Arthritis

A practical guide to getting on with your life

Dr Chris Jenner

howtobooks

Published by How To Books Ltd,
Spring Hill House, Spring Hill Road,
Begbroke, Oxford OX5 1RX,United Kingdom.
Tel: (01865) 375794. Fax: (01865) 379162.
info@howtobooks.co.uk
www.howtobooks.co.uk

How To Books greatly reduce the carbon footprint of their books by sourcing
their typesetting and printing in the UK.

First edition 2011

British Library Cataloguing in Publication Data
A catalogue record for this book is available from the British Library

ISBN 978 1 84528 471 8

Illustrations by Firecatcher
Cover design by Baseline Arts Ltd, Oxford
Produced for How To Books by Deer Park Productions, Tavistock
Typeset by PDQ Typesetting Ltd, Newcastle-under-Lyme, Staffs.
Printed and bound in Great Britain by Bell & Bain Ltd, Glasgow

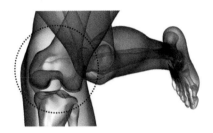

Arthritis

Other self-help guides
by How To Books

Neck and Back Pain
Dr Chris Jenner

Fibromyalgia and Myofascial Pain Syndrome
Dr Chris Jenner

howtobooks

How To Books
Spring Hill House, Spring Hill Road,
Begbroke, Oxford OX5 1RX
info@howtobooks.co.uk
www.howtobooks.co.uk

Contents

Part II Living with Arthritis

Part III Treating and Managing Arthritis

Part IV Understanding Medico-Legal Implications

Preface

Because so many people suffer from arthritis, and so many others know a sufferer personally, this is a condition which many are tempted to treat as trivial. In fact though, arthritis in its many different forms can cause devastation to the lives of those who suffer from it, as well as to those of their families.

Although the term 'arthritis' tends to suggest a single disease, in fact it incorporates a range of more than 100 separate conditions, some of which have certain similarities, and others of which are quite distinct. In this book, I take a look at some of the more and less common forms of the disease, but because the book is aimed at sufferers and their families, you will not find any complex medical explanations, just easy-to-understand descriptions of the conditions themselves, along with their causes and symptoms, information on how they are diagnosed and the treatment options which are available.

This book, however, is not just aimed at providing straightforward medical information, because arthritis is not a condition which touches solely on the physical existence of the sufferer. Like many chronic pain conditions, it frequently affects people at an emotional and psychological level too, impacting on every area of their lives, including their relationships and their work and home lives. It raises challenges and frustrations from every side and can leave those who are caught in its grip feeling helpless and isolated. Being diagnosed with arthritis can literally stir up feelings of grief for a life lost or altered beyond recognition. These are all issues that I have seen time and time again in the many, many patients that I have treated over the years, and yet they are ones which are all too often ignored.

Sadly, the treatment that many people receive for arthritis is what can only be described as one-dimensional. It focuses on traditional pharmaceutical medications which are aimed at tackling pain and other symptoms. Arthritis though, is not a simple disease. It is a highly complex condition which affects sufferers on many different levels and requires a much more sophisticated and multidisciplinary approach.

The fact is that much of the misery of arthritis can be avoided, but all too often those who are diagnosed with the condition are not shown how. No matter whether you or someone close to you has been recently diagnosed with the disease, or whether it has been part of your life for many years, it is my sincere hope that within the pages of this book you will find new hope and the way forward into a happier, more pain-free and more successful life.

Dr Christopher Jenner MB BS, FCRA
London Pain Clinic

Part One

Understanding Arthritis

1

What Is Arthritis?

The word 'arthritis' literally means inflammation of the joints, but rather than referring to a single disease, the term actually covers more than 100 medical conditions which, in different ways and for different reasons, cause pain, stiffness and loss of movement. What all of these conditions have in common, however, is that they affect the musculoskeletal system, and the joints of the body specifically. Another mutual and unfortunate similarity is that none of these conditions are currently curable and most have the propensity to cause immense suffering and impairment to the quality of lives of those who experience their effects.

Arthritis is commonly thought of as a condition which affects only older members of society, and indeed some forms of the condition are not only more prevalent in those over the age of 55, but are responsible for more cases of disability in this age group in developed countries than any other single disease or illness. Other forms of arthritis, however, can develop during the various stages of life and some as early as infancy. As the disease takes hold, the weakness, swelling and instability of the joints which are fairly typical of many forms of the condition can make carrying out even the most basic activities difficult or even impossible, and in some cases can even produce visible deformities which only add to the sufferer's distress.

There are almost 200 separate joints in the human body and arthritis can potentially affect any of these. In many cases, those who suffer from an arthritis-related condition find that more than one joint is affected, with knees, wrists, elbows, hands and hips being some of the most commonly affected areas. The joints of the spine too can fall prey to arthritis and in many cases the disease can become progressively worse and spread from one area of the body to another. Both the severity of the condition and the particular joints affected will do much to determine the extent of pain symptoms, as well as the potential for mobility to become restricted.

Although arthritis is principally a disease which affects muscle and bone, some forms of the condition have much more widespread effects and can, in fact, impact on the entire body. These systemic forms can, for example, cause damage to the body's primary organs such as the heart, lungs, kidneys and even the skin, as well as impairing other bodily systems and functions. Osteoarthritis, which is the most common type of arthritis, however, is restricted to the joints, while the much more serious but widespread rheumatoid arthritis affects the joints, tendons and tissues of the body.

As I have suggested, different forms of arthritis attack the body in different ways. Certain types of the condition, for example, are caused by wear and tear and so typically affect those in the older age groups, whereas others are autoimmune diseases, are caused by infections or viruses, or develop as the result of an excess or depletion of certain substances in the body. Accidents and injuries can also be responsible for certain types of the disease, although it can sometimes be many years before the arthritis becomes apparent.

The different types of arthritis are not equally well understood, and in most cases medical science has yet to discover a definitive cause. There do, however, appear to be certain factors which make certain individuals more susceptible to one form or another of the condition and I will look at these in more detail when I consider age and gender issues in Chapter 2, as well as in Chapter 5 which deals specifically with the potential causes of the disease. Suffice to say for the moment, however, that alongside age and gender, hereditary factors, previous injuries to the joints and obesity all appear to play a part in the onset of the disease in some cases, and that certain other illnesses seem to act as a precursor to certain types of arthritis.

Like many other chronic illnesses and diseases, arthritis is one whose effects are not just felt at a physical level. Pain is an emotional as well as a sensory experience and living with chronic pain, not to mention the sometimes severe restrictions to mobility which many chronic pain conditions also inflict, can have a significant impact on emotional and psychological well-being too. Although there are clear links between these effects, even today some of those in the medical profession fail to take account of them fully and, in treating only physical symptoms, effectively contribute to the patient's suffering as the effects of emotional and psychological distress begin to aggravate physical symptoms and set up a vicious cycle.

As I mentioned in the Preface though, much of the misery which is typically associated with arthritis is, in fact, avoidable, and it is my aim in this book to demonstrate why this is the case and just how sufferers can turn their lives around and experience a much improved quality of life. Education, of course, is at the very foundation of changing things for the better and, in reading what is to follow, you are taking the first vital step forward.

As you will discover as you read on, this book has not been written with the medical expert in mind, but is aimed at those who suffer from arthritis and those whose partners, family members or friends are afflicted with the disease and who wish to learn more about their conditions. As such, you will not be presented with any confusing or unnecessary medical terminology, just straightforward and easily understandable explanations. In fact, although the book does cover all the essentials in terms of the medical side of the condition, it quite deliberately avoids focussing too heavily on this aspect, but rather concentrates on the more 'human' considerations, such as how arthritis can affect the lives of sufferers and those around them and the practical steps that can be taken to minimise those effects.

Having said all of this, however, because arthritis is a disease which affects the joints, it is helpful to understand a little about the make-up of the joints and how they work so that the different forms of the disease make more sense and so that the effects of factors such as stress, exercise and diet can all be better appreciated. To this end, I will begin by offering a brief and simple explanation of the working of the joints, before moving on in the remainder of this chapter to provide an overview of both the effects of arthritis and the prognosis for those who suffer from the condition. You will find much more detailed information relating to each of the latter in Chapter 3 where I consider the main types of the disease.

How Joints Work

The joints in the human body are essentially where two bones meet and connect with one another. The knee joint, for example, is the point of connection of the thigh bone (the femur) and the shin bone (the tibia). Without joints, clearly we would not be able to bend and flex different parts of our bodies and in fact, in order for us to be able to do so efficiently and without causing ourselves any damage, the human anatomy is designed in such a way that we have different types of joints which move in different ways and which allow different degrees and angles of extension. You have probably heard of, for example, ball and socket joints and hinge joints, which are just some of the types to be found in our bodies.

Joints are made up of various components which are all designed to connect the bones and hold them in place, to protect the bones, to allow the joint to move as it should and to join one component to another. In the most common types of joints, known as synovial joints, the ends of the two bones and some of the other components which make the joints work are contained within a fibrous sac called a joint capsule or synovial sac. You can see what the cross-section of a healthy joint looks like in Figure 1.1.

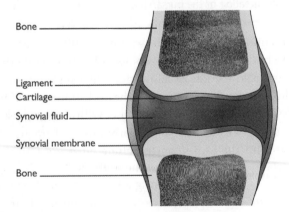

Figure 1.1 Cross-section of a healthy joint

The main components of the joint and what they do are as follows.

- **Cartilage** – cartilage, or articular cartilage, is a tough material which covers the surface of the ends of the bones where they meet. It acts as a cushion to protect the bones and lets the joint work smoothly, but if it is worn away or otherwise caused to degenerate, then the bones can rub directly and painfully against one another.
- **Ligaments** – ligaments are quite short fibrous cords, a bit like elastic bands, which are typically found around the joints and inside the joint capsule. They are attached to each of the bones and they not only hold these together and keep the joint stable, but they also hold the bones in the proper alignment.
- **Synovial sac** – the synovial sac basically encompasses the joint. Within the synovial sac or membrane, the joint cavity is filled with synovial fluid which protects and lubricates the joint as well as providing nourishment to the cartilage.
- **Muscles** – muscles sit outside the synovial sac but lie close to the joints. They are elastic tissues which have the ability to become shorter and longer, so allowing the joint to move.
- **Tendons** – tendons are another type of fibrous cord, but unlike the shorter ligaments which attach bone to bone, these longer cords attach bone to muscle. Tendons have no elasticity like muscles, which is why you hear of tendons 'snapping', but instead they move with the muscle.
- **Bursa** – although the bursa is not actually part of the joint itself, it does sit close by, in between the bone and the muscle. In many ways, it is similar to the synovial sac and it contains a lubricating fluid which helps muscle to move across muscle or bone more easily. You may have heard of the condition known as bursitis which is the inflammation of the bursa.

As I mentioned earlier, there are almost 200 different joints in the human body, all of which can potentially suffer from the effects of wear and tear, the loss of lubrication, deposits of crystals, infection or injury, or develop problems as the body starts attacking itself as is the case with autoimmune disorders. Arthritis is the result of something going wrong with a joint or joints, and frequently with the area around the joints, but precisely what goes wrong depends upon the type of arthritis that the individual is suffering from.

The Effects of Arthritis

The effects of arthritis can vary hugely from person to person and much will depend on the severity of the type of the disease which is experienced, as well as on how long the individual has had the condition. In addition, however, because our responses to pain can be determined by past experiences or, for example, by how our parents taught us to react to it, two people suffering from the same condition at the same level of severity for the same length of time can still experience it in entirely different ways. How well or badly patients accept and deal positively with their condition, meanwhile, can have an enormous impact on the severity of their symptoms.

Broadly speaking, the more common forms of arthritis tend to manifest themselves in the form of:

- Discomfort
- Persistent pain
- Sharp, stabbing pains
- A mixture of aches and pains
- Stiffness
- Restricted range of motion
- Fatigue, and in some cases,
- Swelling and redness of the joints

Other types of the condition, however, can also produce:

- Rashes
- Fever
- Lumps of tissue under the skin
- Loss of appetite
- Weight loss
- Anaemia

Usually, the intensity of arthritis symptoms tends to fluctuate, with sufferers experiencing both good days and bad. In cases where the condition has become chronic, however, and the individual lives in fear of the next bad day, the good days can become extremely difficult to appreciate and the patient's whole life can become consumed with feelings of dread. On the bad days, meanwhile, the pain, lack of mobility and inability to even grip or hold things securely can lead to intense frustration and distress.

Another one of the difficulties associated with arthritis is that the disease can sometimes cause secondary problems. As mobility becomes impaired, exercise becomes more difficult and weight gets harder to lose, so the patient's overall physical condition begins to deteriorate, even to the extent where the individual becomes house-bound and bedridden, and infections such as pneumonia can much more readily take hold. In addition, where mobility becomes an issue, there is a greater risk of falls which can result in fractures and yet further complications. Treating arthritis early and using a holistic approach which not only aims to minimise pain, but also to improve and maintain function and mobility, is vital if the like-lihood of secondary problems is to be reduced.

Aside from the physical effects of arthritis, as I said previously, in its chronic form the condition can also lead to emotional or psy-chological issues, with depression and anxiety often becoming very real side effects of the disease. The combination of intense pain and restricted mobility, along with the enforced changes which can impact on every area of sufferers' lifestyles can leave them strug-gling considerably with their day-to-day lives and feeling hopeless about their futures. Fears of what lies ahead can soon become all-consuming as patients start on the downward spiral towards despair.

For those who do not suffer from arthritis, it can be hard to appreciate just how wide ranging its effects can be. Some signs, such as not being able to pick up or handle things, difficulties with walking or having to give up treasured hobbies may be more obvious, but behind all of these there can be problems with personal and intimate relationships, parenting issues, work issues, financial concerns and even concerns about image which often go unrecognised by the outside world. Frequently, sufferers themselves are taken by surprise at the extent to which their condition impacts on their existence and the way in which it can exacerbate problems which may already have been bubbling away under the surface. A relationship which was beginning to feel the very earliest signs of strain, for example, can suddenly feel overwhelmingly difficult when the pressures of the disease are added.

The Prognosis

At almost any level of severity, arthritis has the potential to affect a person's life in one way or another, and in some cases those effects can be devastating. Even though there is no known cure for the disease at present that does not mean that sufferers cannot still live an active, productive and fulfilling life. In fact, a great deal can be done through the treatment and management of the disease to minimise its impact and restore a reasonable quality of life.

Considerable research has shown that by far the most effective approach to chronic pain conditions such as arthritis are those which are multidisciplinary. While pharmaceutical drugs alone can have positive impacts on levels of pain, they generally do little or nothing to affect mobility and can even cause side effects of their own which detract even further from the sufferer's quality of life. Popping pills in itself can neither teach a patient how to accept their condition or manage their symptoms, nor how to restore any semblance of normality or quality to their existence. It cannot prolong their period of independence, keep them out of a wheel-chair or help them to deal with the effects of their disease on their close personal relationships, their friendships or their work. In many cases, however, doctors' responses to these conditions simply involve prescribing medication and leaving patients to sort the rest out for themselves.

Learning to live happily and successfully with arthritis requires a holistic approach which not only tackles pain and mobility issues directly, but also provides sufferers with practical solutions which allow them to continue their daily lives with minimal disruption. Although some type of medication often does form part of a treatment programme, only when it is combined with other types of therapy, other techniques and other conscious changes to lifestyle will it have maximum effect.

As you can imagine, the prognosis for those who suffer from arthritis varies hugely, irrespective of the type of the condition that they have been diagnosed with. Those whose conditions remain untreated can be doomed to lives of intense pain and misery in which the disease worsens and irreversible effects are experienced. At the other end of the spectrum, however, those who follow a multidisciplinary treatment programme and make a commitment to their own well-being have the potential to live relatively or even wholly pain-free existences with only minimal affects on mobility, and in which attitude and certain changes to lifestyle allow them to take full control of their lives.

2

Arthritis – The Statistics

Figuring out just how many people around the world suffer from arthritis is not a simple task. Not only do different organisations gather and record their statistics using different methodologies, but so too do different organisations in different countries. To make things even more difficult, some cases of the disease occur in episodes rather than being continual and others have no standard definitions. Some countries do not even collect data of their own and so many of the statistics that we see are extrapolated from estimates for other nations. These, however, may not be very accurate because there are those who believe that people in less developed countries are less likely to suffer from the disease due to diet and other lifestyle factors. Having said this, however, arthritis is reported to be the most common cause of disability in the UK and the USA.

It is actually not too difficult to imagine how many people are affected by arthritis, simply because there are few of us who do not know someone with the condition. To give you an idea of how many sufferers we are talking about though, as well as of some statistical evidence of the effects of the disease on society, I have drawn largely on the data published by the highly respected, leading arthritis charity in the UK, Arthritis Care, in a factsheet which was last reviewed in 2007. Unless stated otherwise, the statistics to follow are courtesy of this organisation.

As I said earlier, despite that many people see it as an 'old person's disease', arthritis is no respecter of age. Infants, children, teenagers and adults of all ages can develop different forms of the condition and later on in this chapter you will find some statistics which give an idea of how different age groups are affected, as well as the effects of the condition on the different genders.

UK Incidence

Arthritis is the most common chronic condition in the UK and is believed to affect more than 10 million people in a way which limits their activities. It is even more prevalent than heart and respiratory conditions and, according to a survey conducted in 2001, accounted at that time for 28% of all long-term conditions. Research which was carried out several years ago indicated that around one in every five adults in the country is affected by the disease, but in what is an ageing population, this percentage has almost certainly grown. According to a Scottish study into joint problems, the findings of which were published in 2005, one out of every four consultations with general practitioners (GPs) in the UK was believed to be in relation to arthritis.

Osteoarthritis, which is the most common form of the disease, affected 8.5 million people in the UK according to an Arthritis Care study which was published in 2002. Statistics reported by Arthritis Research UK in November 2008, meanwhile, showed that more than 6 million people in the UK had osteoarthritis in one or both knees and more than 650,000 in one or both hips. There was, however X-ray evidence of the hips being affected in a further 1.5 million people who may not have had any symptoms.

Problems with the knees and hips in general accounted for almost 59,000 primary hip replacements in England and Wales in 2006/7, with 94% of these being required as a result of osteoarthritis. The same year saw more than 62,000 primary knee replacements being carried out in England and Wales, 97% due to the condition, and in Scotland, 6,000 hip replacements and 6,300 knee replacements were done. With the average cost of a hip replacement in the UK amounting to £7,350, that makes the total cost of these operations in the region of £477 million in a single year.

Knee replacement surgery, which perhaps surprisingly costs more than hip replacement surgery, is somewhat of a controversial issue in the UK because obesity is the biggest risk factor for osteoarthritis of the knee and so accounts for the majority of the vast sums of money that are spent on this type of operation. With the somewhat dubious distinction of having the third highest obesity rate in the world at the time of writing, and with obesity being, in nearly every case, preventable, some health authorities in the UK are now refusing to carry out knee replacements unless the patient's body mass index is within certain limits.

Albeit that osteoarthritis of the knee and hip are so common, according to Arthritis Research UK, this form of the disease is most often found in the spine, and their November 2008 report indicated that almost 8.5 million people could have X-ray evidence of the condition in this area, although again, some people may suffer no symptoms at all or may not suffer symptoms which are severe enough to report to their GPs. Other research indicates that around half of all sufferers have X-ray evidence of moderate to severe osteoarthritis in their hands.

Rheumatoid arthritis, meanwhile, was believed by Arthritis Research UK to affect around 400,000 adults in the UK in 2008, with approximately 20,000 new cases being diagnosed in the country each year, up from the 12,000 reported just six years earlier in Arthritis Care's factsheet. In addition, more than 300,000 people are said to visit their GP each year because of ankylosing spondylitis, around 25,000 due to systemic lupus erythematosus and over a quarter of a million because of gout.

As if these statistics were not worrying enough in themselves, Arthritis Care's factsheet, which draws on a range of information sources, points out that:

- 93% of arthritis sufferers have difficulty walking
- 37% can only walk a few steps
- 72% meet the legal definition of disabled as laid down by the Disability Discrimination Act 1995
- 87% of those with arthritis or joint pain are not under the care of a rheumatologist or orthopaedic surgeon
- 81% of people are in constant pain or are limited in terms of their ability to perform everyday tasks
- 80% suffer sleep disturbances due to being woken by pain which is at its worst during the night

Notably, however, the organisation's own studies have found that 57% of sufferers of osteoarthritis use exercise to help manage their conditions, something which one must assume they do because they feel its beneficial effects. In addition, those who suffer from osteoarthritis and are employed experience pain less frequently.

In terms of the costs to society of arthritis, the condition is responsible for:

- A spend of £5.7 billion per year (2008 figure)
- The loss of 10 million working days (in 2006/7)
- The highest number of claims for Disability Living Allowance
- Over 90% of all GP referrals to physiotherapists
- 6 million people providing unpaid care in the UK

US Incidence

Although some sources show the prevalence of arthritis in the USA as being as high as almost 70 million, a report produced by the American College of Rheumatology in 2008, along with numerous other reliable studies, indicates that just over 46 million adults, or more than 21% of the adult population of America, suffered from 'self-reported, doctor-diagnosed' arthritis. While 1.3 million adults were believed to have rheumatoid arthritis, anywhere between 600,000 and 2.4 million were thought to suffer from spondyloarthritis, between 161,000 and 322,000 from systemic lupus erythematosus, 49,000 from systemic sclerosis and between 400,000 and 3.1 million from Sjögren's syndrome.

As elsewhere, including the UK, osteoarthritis is the most common form of the disease in the USA, with nearly 27 million Americans suffering from the condition. For a number of years, the USA has held the top ranking in the world for obesity and in 2006 one source estimated that nearly 3.5 million Americans would need a knee replacement.

Estimates in terms of cases of rheumatoid arthritis in the USA dropped in the years from 1990 to 2005 from 2.1 million to 1.3 million and the average age of diagnosis has increased steadily over time. It is believed, however, that around half of Americans who suffer from the disease become so disabled by the condition that they are no longer able to work 10 years after being diagnosed.

The American Arthritis Foundation reported in 2004 that the direct and indirect costs associated with the various types of the disease amounted to $86.2 billion, only 3% of which related to drugs. In the same year, labour force participation was reduced by 20% for men and 25% for women as a result of the condition.

Again, the worrying thing in relation to US sufferers is that 57% of those who have been diagnosed with arthritis are not receiving treatment. The situation does not look set to get any better either, with the number of sufferers being expected to rise by a further 40% by the year 2030 and 25% of Americans with the condition becoming forced to limit their daily activities.

Global Incidence

Elsewhere in the world, it has to be said that the picture does not look very much less bleak. Figures published in 2004 suggested that when looked at as a whole, Europe was at that time home to more than 100 million arthritis sufferers and a further study indicated that more people in Europe are affected by the disease than by any other chronic condition. As in the UK, around one in every four visits to European doctors is related to the condition.

In Australia, meanwhile, 2004 statistics showed that 3.4 million people, or 16.7% of the population has the disease, with 60% of these being of working age. The total cost to the country in that year amounted to $19.25 billion in direct and indirect costs.

Over in Asia, while 5% of the Japanese population or 6 million people suffer from arthritis, in Southern China the figure jumps to 22%. In this area, the incidence of gout is significantly higher than in other parts of China and this form of the condition is responsible for affecting as many as 28% of young people.

South Africa, meanwhile, not only has the issue of arthritis in general to deal with, with one in seven in the country suffering from the condition, but also the fact that 2004 reports indicated only 30 rheumatology consultants for a population of 40 million people. That is just one consultant per 1.3 million people. In addition, with AIDS being a particular problem in this part of the world, a variant of reactive arthritis which is AIDS related has been emerging and is causing serious concern.

The Gender Issue

In common with certain other medical conditions, arthritis does not affect both genders equally. Studies conducted in countries around the world have consistently found that the disease overall is far more common in women than it is in men. In the UK, for example, the Focus on Health report which was published by the Office of National Statistics in 2006 showed that the condition is twice as prevalent in women as it is in men. Of the hip and knee replacement operations carried out in England and Wales in 2006/7, 60% and 57% respectively of surgeries were done on female patients. The National Arthritis Data Workgroup in the USA, meanwhile, estimated in their 2005 study that more than 60% of arthritis sufferers in the country were women.

When the most common different types of arthritis are looked at separately, much the same picture emerges, with only a few notable exceptions. Osteoarthritis, by far the most common type, affects women more frequently than men and is largely responsible for the greater prevalence overall in the female sex. Rheumatoid arthritis, meanwhile, is believed to strike two to four times more women and Arthritis Research UK showed in their November 2008 report that systemic lupus erythematosus is more common in females by a ratio of 7:1. One of the biggest exceptions is in relation to gout, which not only affects more men, but is also more prevalent amongst older males.

Not surprisingly, the gender difference is one which is of great interest to doctors and scientists and I will look at some of the theories which have been put forward as to why more women suffer from most forms of the disease than men when I consider the causes of arthritis in Chapter 5. Irrespective of the possible causes, however, one thing which is evident from the various studies which have been carried out is that women seem to experience greater suffering as a result of the condition than men, not just in a physiological sense, but also in an emotional one.

Pain, as I have explained, is an entirely personal thing which is experienced differently by every single individual, but there do appear to be real and substantial variations between the sexes. In the case of arthritis, these do not just manifest themselves in terms of the severity of the pain experienced, but also in the extent to which and the ways in which men and women cope with pain and their behaviours in the face of a chronic pain condition.

From a physical perspective, hormones, chromosomes or differences in immune responses between the sexes might well account for the fact that women typically report more severe symptoms and greater levels of disability than men. In addition, because a woman naturally has less physical strength than a man, any condition which causes a further loss of strength is likely to have a greater impact on her functional status than it would on that of her male counterpart. Effectively, a woman's baseline strength is lower and so even though she may suffer the same loss of strength as a man, it will leave her feeling far more depleted. What is interesting, however, is that some studies have shown that even when these more severe symptoms are taken into account, women use more strategies to cope with their pain and are better at regulating the emotions which are experienced as a result of pain. For example, men typically suffer more intensely from negative feelings, moods and emotions in the wake of painful episodes than women do.

Another difference which is evident between the sexes is in the course of the disease. In the case of rheumatoid arthritis, for instance, the disease appears to progress much more rampantly in women in its earlier stages when the condition is naturally at its most aggressive. The mortality rate for this type of arthritis, however, is higher in younger males, although it does increase rapidly in women with age.

The Age Issue

Although the incidence of the most common type of arthritis, osteoarthritis, as well as some other forms of the condition, does increase with age, it would be most misleading to describe arthritis generally as an 'old person's disease'. In fact, some types of the condition are unique to youngsters and of the estimated 46 million arthritis sufferers in the USA, almost two-thirds are below the age of 65. In reality, no age group is immune to the disease.

In 2006, the Royal College of General Practitioners – Birmingham Research Unit reported that while one in every ten people between the ages of 15 and 24 visit their GP each year with arthritis and related conditions, this figure rises to one in three in the over-75 age group. The authors of the 2004 report on the North Staffordshire Osteoarthritis Project, meanwhile, noted that more than one-third of the population over the age of 50 experiences pain which interferes with their normal activities.

While the chances of becoming a sufferer, particularly of osteoarthritis, do therefore increase with age, osteoarthritis is not believed by many to be an inevitable part of ageing in the same way that developing wrinkles or having our hair turn grey is however. Rather than just being the result of normal wear and tear on the body, it is thought that other factors such as injuries and abnormal ways of moving are largely responsible for the wearing of the joints and the subsequent pain and stiffness. Whatever leads to the development of the condition though, because age is a relevant factor and because we live in an ageing population, the number of sufferers is likely to continue growing into the future.

As I mentioned previously, the average age of diagnosis for rheumatoid arthritis has increased steadily over time, but this condition can appear at any age, although the average age of onset is generally between 25 and 50. Gout, on the other hand, is more prevalent in older males, with an estimated 90% of cases occurring in men over the age of 40 and the peak age being around 75.

In the case of the juvenile forms of arthritis, a UK estimate in 2008 suggested that 1–2 children out of every 1,000 are affected by juvenile chronic arthritis, while the prevalence of juvenile idiopathic arthritis is estimated to be around 6 in 10,000, with one new case of the disease appearing in every 10,000 children per year. Based on research carried out in 2001, Arthritis Care reported in their factsheet which was last reviewed in 2007 that a total of 12,000 children in the UK suffer from juvenile idiopathic arthritis. Other estimates put the number of individuals under the age of 25 in the UK who suffer from some type of arthritis at around 27,000. In America, meanwhile, juvenile idiopathic arthritis and other rheumatic conditions are said to affect approximately 294,000 children between infancy and the age of 17.

The Race Issue

Research carried out by the National Arthritis Data Workgroup in the USA in 2005 indicates that, overall, the prevalence in white people and African Americans in the country is similar, but that it is lower for Hispanics. In the case of osteoarthritis, however, more African Americans than white people are believed to be affected and in the case of gout, older African American males seem to be more prone than older white or Hispanic males. The results of the National Health Interview Survey 2002, 2003 and 2006 published by the Centers for Disease Control and Prevention, however, also take into account American Indians and Native Alaskans, and it is this group which shows the highest prevalence of arthritis across all types of the condition.

Although I do not intend to address the effects of racial differences in relation to arthritis specifically in this book, it is perhaps worth mentioning that there are those who believe that the reason why there are disparities across different racial groups is because of differences in diet. One source, for example, notes that certain tribes in India enjoy exceptionally good health and low prevalence rates of diseases such as arthritis and osteoporosis, and that these things are attributed to the healthy food that these people grow and eat. As diet is, of course, a very important factor in terms of maintaining healthy joints and bones, there may well be a solid foundation to this theory. In addition, as there are strong links between obesity and osteoarthritis in particular, and because obesity tends to be less of a problem outside the developed nations, this too could explain why the disease is less prevalent in these populations.

3

Types of Arthritis

As I described at the start of this book, rather than referring to a single disease, arthritis is an umbrella term which takes into account more than 100 different conditions, all of which affect the joints or the areas surrounding the joints of the body. Often there is a fine line between what experts consider to be a form of arthritis and conditions which are very closely related to the disease, meaning that different sources separate them according to different criteria. There are those, for example, who include fibromyalgia as a type of arthritis, despite the fact that the former does not directly affect the joints and does not cause any physiological damage to them. As some types of arthritis present with very similar symptoms and as some co-exist with fibromyalgia, however, it is easy to see why this confusion occurs.

The criteria that I have used in this book to separate what might be thought of as 'true' arthritic conditions from related medical conditions are largely based on whether or not the primary effects of the disease are on the joints or the areas surrounding the joints. In this chapter, therefore, the conditions that I have chosen to discuss are those where this is the case, whereas in Chapter 4 the ones that you will read about are those which are closely related to arthritis, which frequently give rise to the condition or which can stem from the disease. Starting with the two most common types of arthritis, osteoarthritis and rheumatoid arthritis, the remainder of this chapter is arranged so that the different diseases appear in alphabetical order.

Osteoarthritis

Understanding the Condition

Osteoarthritis, which is often referred to as degenerative arthritis or degenerative joint disease, is the form of arthritis which most people associate with ageing and it is caused by the degeneration of the cartilage, the tough material which protects the ends of the bones where they meet and form the joint. Although it occurs much more frequently in older people, as I mentioned previously, it is not an inevitable part of the ageing process and it can in fact afflict people of any age. Generally, the disease develops gradually over time.

The cartilage which covers the ends of the bones normally acts as a cushion, as well as helping to distribute force and weight evenly when pressure is put on the joint. As you can see from Figure 3.1, what happens in osteoarthritis is that the cartilage begins to break down, becoming rough, brittle and weak, and the body tries to compensate for this by causing the bone underneath it to become thicker and by developing bony growths called osteophytes around the edge of the affected joint. At the same time, the synovial sac or membrane which surrounds the joint also becomes thicker and the space inside the sac where the synovial fluid is contained becomes smaller. As the cartilage degenerates, so the ligaments and tendons start to become stretched and painful. Over time and as the condition worsens, however, bits of cartilage then begin to break away from the bone altogether so that the exposed ends of the bones rub together and cause what is typically severe pain. The combination of all of these factors can not only alter the shape of the joint or make it appear enlarged, but it can also force the bones out of alignment and cause instability in the joint as well as deformity.

Osteoarthritis mainly occurs in the weight-bearing joints of the body, with the hips, knees, feet, neck and lower back being some of the areas most commonly affected. The fingers and the base of the thumbs are also particularly prone to the condition, but in fact almost any joint in the body can be affected. Symptoms tend to develop slowly and worsen over time and typically include some or all of the following:

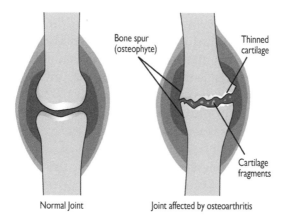

Figure 3.1 Comparison of a healthy joint with one affected by osteoarthritis

- Pain in the joint either during or after use
- Pain in the joint after periods of inactivity
- Pain in the joint after repetitive use
- Joint stiffness, especially first thing in the morning and following periods of inactivity
- Loss of flexibility
- Tenderness when pressure is applied to the joint
- A grating sensation when the joint is used
- Creaking of the affected joints
- A knobbly appearance to the joint where bone spurs or osteophytes have developed
- Swelling of the joints and/or warmth in and around the affected area

The pain associated with osteoarthritis varies from person to person and might range from mild to severe or be continuous or spasmodic. Often it is described as feeling like a deep ache and whilst in some cases patients find that the pain lessens or disappears entirely during rest or sleep, in others it does not abate at all. Commonly, sufferers complain that the pain feels worse later on in the day. Sometimes, symptoms will even disappear quite inexplicably for years, only to return just as mysteriously at a later date.

The stiffness of the joints that most patients experience tends to be alleviated when the joint is moved, although as movement becomes progressively more difficult, so the danger of the condition causing disability increases. Even normal day-to-day activities such as travelling in a car or sitting through a film at the cinema can make the joints feel as though they have seized up, not to mention cause severe pain.

Unlike some of the other forms of arthritis, osteoarthritis is limited to the joints themselves and the area immediately surrounding them. Although it does not affect the organs of the body, however, in the case of osteoarthritis of the spine, for example, the wearing away of cartilage (in the form of the intervertebral discs) and the overgrowth of bone can lead to nerves becoming trapped or pinched and resulting pain, as well as numbness, weakness, tingling sensations and difficulties in walking. In cases where bony growths appear in the upper part of the spine in the neck these can even press against the oesophagus and cause difficulties in swallowing.

Because the hands are on show more than any other part of the body, when osteoarthritis affects the fingers, it is here that the disease is usually most noticeable. In some cases it is just the joints towards the ends of the fingers which are affected by additional bony growth which makes the joints look enlarged (known as Heberden's nodes), whilst in others it is the middle joints (bony enlargements here are called Bouchard's nodes) or indeed both sets of joints. Despite the fact that osteoarthritis of the hands looks extremely painful because of the deformity that it causes, there is not always pain associated with the condition, although typically there are restrictions to the movement of the joints which can make it extremely difficult for sufferers to grip or hold objects. In some cases, such as when the individual is trying to pick up a pan or kettle full of boiling water or something fairly heavy, this can make carrying out normal daily tasks quite hazardous.

Osteoarthritis which affects the joint at the base of the big toe often leads to the formation of a bunion, which is effectively just an enlargement of the bone or tissue around the joint. The bump which appears to the side of the joint not only causes a deformity and often feels swollen and tender, but it can also cause the big toe to turn inwards, causing footwear to become ill-fitting and discomfort to result. As both this type of osteoarthritis and osteoarthritis of the hands have been found to affect the female line in certain families, it is believed that they may have a genetic cause.

Generally speaking, as osteoarthritis progresses, joints become more and more difficult to move and eventually it becomes impossible for them to be bent or straightened fully. Where the ligaments which support the joint become stretched, the joint too becomes unstable, making normal movements such as standing, walking and climbing stairs not only extremely difficult and painful, but also risky in terms of causing further damage. The extent of the degeneration of the joints in osteoarthritis can though, be misleading when considered in relation to the severity of symptoms. In some cases, X-rays show evidence of considerable damage but the patient only experiences low levels of pain or stiffness. In others, however, the degeneration only appears to be slight, but the individual is severely debilitated by his or her symptoms.

Risk Factors for Developing the Condition

The underlying cause of osteoarthritis has not, as yet, been identified, and in most cases the reasons why the disease is triggered in certain individuals are unknown. There are, however, certain risk factors which make it more likely for certain groups of people to suffer from it. Being female is one of the greatest risk factors, as is being overweight, but injury to a joint (albeit that the condition might not manifest itself until many years after the injury was sustained) or infection of a joint can also trigger the disease. In some, although certainly not all cases, having a family member who suffers or suffered from the disease also seems to lead to a predisposition towards the condition and osteoarthritis can also develop as a result of another illness or disease. As repeated stress on a single joint or multiple joints can also be a factor in osteoarthritis, those whose work involves repetitive movements can also be at risk. In cases where the trigger for the disease lies undiscovered, the condition is referred to as primary osteoarthritis, and where another condition acts as the trigger, it is known as secondary osteoarthritis.

As well as being responsible for the development of heart disease and other illnesses of the body, obesity is a highly significant factor in relation to osteoarthritis, particularly in terms of affecting the hips and the knees. Excess body weight exerts a mechanical stress on the joints in general and on the cartilage in the knees in particular, which in turn leads to degeneration. This is why weight lifters, who typically carry excess weight in their upper bodies, have frequently been found to develop the disease fairly early on in life.

Footballers, meanwhile, are just some of those who are at greater risk of developing osteoarthritis of the knee and hip as a result of repeated injuries. Former Arsenal goalkeeper Bob Wilson is just one example of a football player who has suffered decades of pain in the wake of the punishment that both knees and hips sustained during his heyday. X-rays taken 27 years on showed that the cartilage had almost completely worn away, leaving bone rubbing against bone, and that he had been suffering from osteoarthritis for years. With two hip replacements now behind him, at the time of writing he is currently awaiting a knee replacement too.

It is not just professional sportsmen and women who are at risk of injuries which might lead to osteoarthritis though. One study has shown that half of all those who attend a gym at least three times a week or who take part in equivalent levels of exercise have sustained at least one sporting injury. When you bear in mind that one in every two people who sustain a ligament or cartilage tear to the knee develop osteoarthritic pain and disability within 20 years of being diagnosed with the original injury, and that those who have cartilage damage to the knees are five times more likely to develop the disease, there is clearly a great risk to a high proportion of the general population and a great need for anyone who sustains an injury to a joint to seek treatment and advice in the immediate aftermath of an injury or, better still, to take care to avoid being injured in the first place.

This does not, of course, mean that it is advisable to give up on all forms of exercise because it is not the exercise in itself which causes the problem, as is evidenced by the case of long-distance runners. This particular group of athletes has been shown to be at no increased risk of osteoarthritis despite the continual pounding that their limbs take, and this presumably has much to do with the fact that they are much less likely to incur injuries such as those sustained in football or rugby tackles. While you may not of course wish to change your sporting activities in favour of something safer, it is, however, important to take great care to avoid potential injuries if you are involved in sports where any kind of physical contact is likely to cause damage to the joints.

As Bob Wilson would no doubt confirm, osteoarthritis of the knees and hips can cause excruciating pain and immobility. The progressive degeneration of the cartilage in the knees, however, can also lead to an outward curvature of the knees so that the sufferer begins to look bowlegged. The patient may also develop a limp as the result of the damage, which worsens over time as even more of the cartilage degenerates. It is in these more severe cases that total knee replacement surgery is typically required.

As I have mentioned, obesity and injuries are not the only things which can lead to secondary osteoarthritis, and the following are just some of the other triggers:

- Surgery which is carried out on the joints can trigger their degeneration
- Structural abnormalities of the joints which are present at birth (known as congenital abnormalities) can lead to mechanical wear and damage to cartilage
- Gout and pseudogout, themselves different forms of arthritis which are caused by the formation of certain types of crystal deposits in the joints can, in addition, lead to secondary osteoarthritis
- Diseases which cause inflammation, including rheumatoid arthritis
- Certain inherited diseases which cause damage to the cartilage such as haemochromatosis, hyperparathyroidism and Wilson's disease which affect how the body stores iron, calcium and copper respectively
- Bone disorders which affect the joints
- Growth hormone disorders

Diagnosis

The diagnosis of osteoarthritis is usually made based on the presentation of symptoms and X-ray evidence, as there is no blood test which can identify its presence. The deformity of the joints of the fingers, as well as the formation of a bunion at the joint at the base of the big toe, of course, also give doctors considerable clues that the disease is affecting these areas.

Treatment

Once the disease has been diagnosed, the aim of treatment is to reduce the levels of pain that patients experience in the affected joint(s), as well as working to improve and maintain joint function and mobility, as there is no cure for the condition. Painkilling medications and anti-inflammatory drugs may be prescribed, but exercise and various types of physical therapies are also extremely important parts of a comprehensive treatment programme. As we have seen, in very severe cases, surgery may be required, which could include total joint replacement.

Because osteoarthritis affects so many people and because the costs to society of treating the condition, not to mention the costs in terms of lost work days and productivity, are so considerable, much research is ongoing to discover what causes it and to develop medications which can either protect the cartilage from degeneration or slow down the progression of the disease. In addition, it is possible that surgical techniques which involve the patient's own cartilage being grown in a laboratory and being used to patch the end of the affected bone(s) could be developed to help osteoarthritis patients. Early research seems to indicate that certain existing drugs, such as doxycycline and tetracycline, seem to slow the progression of the disease and studies are also looking into whether glucosamine or chondroitin improves or protects the quality of cartilage in osteoarthritic joints. In both cases, however, further research is required to establish whether these might constitute effective treatments for the condition, as well as to determine any side effects that they might cause.

Although osteoarthritis is a progressive disease, it is also one which can, to some degree at least, effectively run its course and settle down naturally. While joints can end up looking rather knobbly, sometimes by the time this stage is reached, levels of pain are much less intense and sufferers are able to carry out most of their everyday tasks. Usually, however, there is some residual degree of disability. Using a multidisciplinary approach to treatment, however, the impact of the disease can be minimised from the point of diagnosis onwards.

Rheumatoid Arthritis

Understanding the Condition

Unlike osteoarthritis, which is more about the mechanical wearing away of the cartilage in the joints, rheumatoid arthritis is what is known as an autoimmune disease, which basically means that the body's own immune system attacks the body instead of defending it. The reason why this happens is not currently known and consequently there is no cure for the disease, which is normally diagnosed via a blood test.

Rheumatoid arthritis is an inflammatory form of arthritis and is the most serious of the common types of the disease. It affects around 1% of the population in the USA and roughly the same in the UK, and is serious enough that it can shorten the sufferer's normal life expectancy, particularly in cases where it is not diagnosed and treated early. Although it can affect people of all ages, including children and the elderly, most often it strikes those between the ages of 40 and 60, with two to three times more women being diagnosed with the condition than men.

When the immune system attacks the joints in rheumatoid arthritis, it is the synovial membrane or synovial sac which is primarily affected, not only by becoming inflamed and thickened, but also by producing excess synovial fluid. In addition, however, inflammation occurs in the bursae (the small sacs of fluid which sit between the bone and the muscle and allow the muscles to move smoothly over one another and over bone) and the tendon sheaths (the tubes inside which the tendons move). As is illustrated in Figure 3.2, not only is the joint itself damaged, but over time the cartilage and the bone can also be affected so that secondary osteoarthritis develops. Almost any joint in the body can be affected by rheumatoid arthritis, but often the same joint on both sides of the body is attacked and the disease typically impacts on multiple joints.

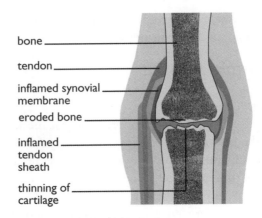

bone

tendon

inflamed synovial
membrane

eroded bone

inflamed
tendon
sheath

thinning of
cartilage

Figure 3.2 Joint affected by rheumatoid arthritis

The most common symptoms of rheumatoid arthritis are pain, stiffness and swelling in the affected joints and the muscles surrounding them, often accompanied by redness and tenderness. As with osteoarthritis, most patients report that the stiffness feels worse in the mornings and after periods of inactivity. In addition to these symptoms, however, patients with rheumatoid arthritis frequently experience:

- Fatigue
- Energy loss
- Lack of appetite and corresponding weight loss
- Low-grade fever

Aside from the extreme pain and loss of mobility that typically comes with rheumatoid arthritis, one of the other things which makes the disease particularly difficult to live with is its unpredictable nature. In common with certain other illnesses such as fibromyalgia, rheumatoid arthritis is normally characterised by periods of remission and flare-ups. During remissions when the disease becomes inactive, inflammation subsides, symptoms disappear and the individual feels generally well. When disease activity starts up anew and a flare-up occurs, however, they are once again returned to a state where they are in considerable pain and where mobility is severely restricted. As remissions can last for weeks, months or even years and can occur quite spontaneously, in addition to being a result of treatment, sufferers can often feel as though they are on an emotional rollercoaster, living not only with the dread of the next flare-up, but of course with the devastating impacts when it does happen.

Rheumatoid arthritis normally develops gradually and often the first symptoms are felt in the small joints in the hands, wrists and feet. Knees and shoulders, however, can also be affected in the earlier stages of the disease. Even the simplest of daily activities such as opening jars or turning doorknobs can become extremely difficult during periods when the disease is active, and those who feel the effects in the larger, weight-bearing joints of the body can experience severe pain when walking, trying to get in and out of cars and so on, and it is not uncommon for climbing stairs to become altogether impossible.

As the inflammation caused by rheumatoid arthritis becomes chronic, the cartilage which covers the ends of the bones can begin to erode and the bones themselves, as well as the muscles, can start to weaken. Not only can this compromise function and mobility, but it can also result in the deformity which is sometimes characteristic of osteoarthritis.

Rheumatoid arthritis does not only confine itself to the joints, however. As a systemic disease (one which affects the whole body rather than just localised areas), it can also cause problems with the skin, blood vessels, lungs and eyes, and occasionally with the heart, brain and even the cells of the immune system itself. Inflammation of the blood vessels, which is known as vasculitis, can not only cause changes to the skin, including painless red or purple-coloured patches which most often appear on the arms and legs, and areas of what look like small reddish black spots (which are painful) around the finger and toenails, but it can also affect the nerves. When the organ systems of the body are affected this can result in internal bleeding, strokes, breathing difficulties and chest pain, as well as redness and pain in the eyes and even loss of vision. Thankfully, however, complications which arise in areas of the body outside of the joints are relatively uncommon, although when they do occur, both men and women are equally likely to be affected.

One effect of rheumatoid arthritis which is seen more commonly in men than women is rheumatoid nodules. Characterised by firm, rubbery lumps under the skin, rheumatoid nodules are found in around 25% of cases of the disease and usually in those who suffer the most chronically and severely. The nodules, which can be pea-sized or even quite considerably bigger, typically appear in areas which are frequently exposed to pressure, such as the elbows, fingers, heels and the back of the head. In some cases they feel 'fixed' under the surface of the skin, whilst in others they are moveable.

Although rheumatoid nodules are not normally troublesome to those who are affected by them, in cases where they appear for example on the heels or the soles of the feet and make walking extremely difficult and painful, they may require treatment in the form of surgery or the injection of steroids to shrink them. Problems can also occur when the skin covering the nodules begins to break down, leaving sores which are open to infection. Wherever possible, however, surgery tends to be avoided, both because it increases the risk of infection and because the nodules tend to reappear almost immediately in places which are exposed to pressure. Despite generally not causing any physical ill-effects, of course rheumatoid nodules do represent a type of deformity and so can still be distressing for sufferers in non-physical ways.

As is the case with most of the different forms of arthritis, the effects of rheumatoid arthritis can vary enormously from one person to the next, although estimates do suggest that some 40% of working sufferers in the UK lose their jobs within five years of being diagnosed with the condition, and that in 75% of these cases, the reasons are as a direct result of the disease. Just over 14%, meanwhile, are said to give up work within one year of diagnosis, which clearly indicates just how debilitating rheumatoid arthritis can be.

Treatment

Despite there being no cure for this form of arthritis, treatment can be highly effective in terms of relieving symptoms, improving and maintaining mobility and ensuring minimal effects on the sufferer's overall quality of life. Although joint replacement surgery is an option in some cases, this is rarely one which is taken up, and only then if there is a danger that the sufferer will lose overall function. Instead, a range of different medications can be used to tackle both pain and inflammation and there are even those which are aimed at slowing the course of the disease. In addition, various types of physical therapy can not only help considerably with mobility issues and in ensuring the most efficient use of the joints so that they do not suffer further damage, but they can also be pain relieving in themselves.

Education about the disease is an important factor which many treatment programmes leave out altogether. In fact though, greater understanding not only helps to promote acceptance and alleviate fear and stress, but it also allows patients to make any necessary adjustments to their lifestyles which will help them to carry on as normal. Even simple things like being aware of special gadgets which make it easier to carry out simple daily tasks or learning how to pace him or herself can make the world of difference to a sufferer's quality of life and help to avoid the periods of frustration which are typically experienced when the disease is active.

Ankylosing Spondylitis

Understanding the Condition

Although many forms of arthritis typically cause damage to a variety of different joints in the body, ankylosing spondylitis is a spinal condition in which the bones, ligaments, tendons and muscles of the back are affected. It is an inflammatory form of arthritis which, according to different reports, affects anywhere between two and three or five times as many men as women. Most often diagnosed in young people in their 20s and 30s, it is thought to occur in 2–5 adults out of every 1,000, 10% of whom could be at risk of long-term disability.

The term 'ankylosing spondylitis' derives from the Greek words meaning 'bent' and 'spine', but in medical terminology 'ankylosing' is used to mean 'stiffening' and 'spondylitis' to mean inflammation of the spine. The condition, therefore, is one in which inflammation of the spinal joints causes them to stiffen.

As can be seen from Figure 3.3, the spine is made up of a series or column of interlocking bones which are known as vertebrae. There are 24 in total, seven of which make up the cervical spine (the part of the spine which runs from the base of the skull down through the neck), 12 of which are situated in the thoracic area (the middle section of the spine) and 5 of which make up the lumbar spine in the lower back and extend downwards towards the sacro-iliac joint and the coccyx.

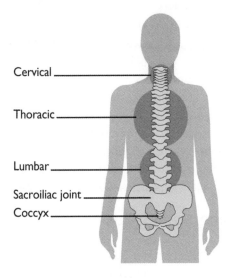

Cervical

Thoracic

Lumbar

Sacroiliac joint

Coccyx

Figure 3.3 The configuration of the human spine

In all, there are 110 separate joints in the spine and these and the spinal vertebrae are supported by muscles, ligaments and tendons which permit and control the movement of the back. What happens in ankylosing spondylitis is that the joints and the structures which support them become inflamed and this inflammation not only causes pain, but also creates stiffness. As Figure 3.4 illustrates, in the body's attempt to heal itself and as the inflammation subsides, new vertical bony outgrowths are formed which can eventually fuse the vertebrae together and make the spine, or at least parts of it, completely inflexible. When this happens, although pain symptoms can sometimes disappear completely, not only can there be considerable restrictions to mobility, but the spine also becomes more vulnerable to fractures.

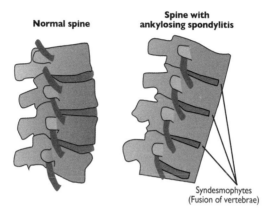

Normal spine

Spine with ankylosing spondylitis

Syndesmophytes
(Fusion of vertebrae)

Figure 3.4 Fusion of the spine caused by ankylosing spondylitis

Ankylosing spondylitis can affect any area of the spine, although it tends to be more common in the lumbar (lower back) and cervical (neck) areas. Particularly in cases where treatment is delayed and significant fusion of the vertebrae occurs it can lead to changes in the normal curvature of the spine and resulting deformity.

The first signs and symptoms of ankylosing spondylitis are generally as a result of the initial inflammation. In the lumbar area of the spine, this typically causes what can be quite severe lower back pain which may spread into the buttocks, hips and the backs of the thighs on one or both sides of the body. Stiffness in the joints normally feels worse first thing in the morning or after periods of inactivity and both pain and stiffness tend to be alleviated by exercise so that the symptoms improve as the day goes on.

Where the mid section of the spine, or the thoracic region, is affected by ankylosing spondylitis, it is the joints which connect the ribs to the vertebrae which become inflamed. Chest pain is one of the most common symptoms, but if the condition progresses to the stage where the joints become stiff or fused, breathing can become more difficult and if the sufferer contracts a cold or respiratory problem, they may find it harder to recover. In the cervical area, meanwhile, pain in the neck and/or shoulders is often the first sign of the condition.

Whichever part of the spine is affected by ankylosing spondylitis, fatigue is often one of the symptoms. In some cases this is caused directly by the activity of the disease itself, whereas in others it is the stress and depression which often accompany the condition that cause the sufferer to feel extremely tired. A feeling of being generally unwell, low-grade fever and weight loss may also be experienced, but generally these symptoms, as well as the pain and stiffness, tend to come and go and vary from mild to severe.

Although ankylosing spondylitis is a condition which starts in the spine, it can progress so that it affects not only other joints in the body such as the shoulders, hips, knees and ankles, but also some of the organs. Inflammation in the valves of the heart, as well as problems with the lungs and kidneys can develop, although these symptoms are relatively uncommon. It is also estimated that as many as 25% of sufferers experience eye problems in the form of iritis. This condition causes inflammation of the coloured part of the eye (the iris), with pain and redness being the result. Rarely does it lead to problems with vision, but it does need to be treated as quickly as possible nevertheless.

The definitive cause of ankylosing spondylitis is not fully understood, but there do appear to be certain genetic links which suggest that some people may be more likely to develop the condition. The genetic marker known as human leukocyte antigen B27 (HLA-B27), for example, has been found to be present in most sufferers, but as most people who carry this gene do not actually develop the condition, clearly it cannot be responsible for being the only cause. Because the gene can be passed down through the generations, however, those who have parents or siblings with ankylosing spondylitis are estimated to be three times more likely to develop the condition than those who do not have a close family member who is a sufferer.

Diagnosis
Diagnosing ankylosing spondylitis is normally achieved using blood tests which are aimed at identifying the presence of inflam-

mation in the joints, as well as through X-rays, magnetic resonance imaging (MRI) scans or ultrasound scans. These latter tests are designed to pick up damage to the joints, changes such as the formation of new bone and inflammation of the joint tissues.

Treatment

Although there is no cure for ankylosing spondylitis, like some other forms of inflammatory arthritis, the disease can spontaneously go into remission or be forced into remission through treatment, so that sufferers experience few or no symptoms for what can be long periods of time. In more severe cases, surgery may be required to replace badly damaged joints such as knees or hips, or to straighten a spine which has become bent. These cases are relatively rare, however, and most patients can be treated very effectively using conservative treatments.

Alongside the use of pain-killing and anti-inflammatory drugs or corticosteroids, physical therapies and exercise are very important elements of a multidisciplinary treatment programme which is aimed at restoring and maintaining mobility in the spine and other affected joints, as well as at increasing muscle strength. Addressing posture too is vital if the impact of the disease is to be minimised. As every case is unique, however, treatment programmes must be individually tailored to suit each patient, and monitoring of progress and adjustment of programmes is essential if the most beneficial results are to be achieved.

Although ankylosing spondylitis is a chronic condition, it rarely causes severe disability, especially if it is managed properly. Most patients are still able to live full and productive lives without the need for surgery.

Fungal Arthritis

Understanding the Condition

Fungal arthritis, which is also known as mycotic arthritis, is the infection of the joint by a fungus. As the human body is normally quite resistant to fungal infection, this is a very rare form of arthritis which tends to affect those whose immune system is compromised for some reason.

The fungi which are most often responsible for fungal arthritis include blastomycosis, candidiasis, cryptococcosis, histoplasmosis and sporotrichosis, and any of these can affect bone or joint tissue. Like septic arthritis, this form of the disease can be found in artificial joints as well as formerly healthy ones and in some cases only one joint is affected, whereas in others the disease can affect multiple joints.

Sometimes, the fungal infection which affects the joints in fungal arthritis spreads from organs such as the lungs where fungal spores are breathed in, but it can also be introduced into the body via:

- Surgical procedures
- Injections into the joints
- Intravenous drug use
- Cuts and scrapes

As most of the fungi responsible for causing the disease can be found in soil, moss, decaying vegetation, bird droppings and hay, those who regularly handle these materials can be at greater risk of infection, but equally, so are those who:

- Have weakened immune systems
- Are undergoing chemotherapy
- Have AIDS
- Use intravenous drugs
- Use medications which suppress the immune system

The large weight-bearing joints of the body tend to be more susceptible to fungal arthritis, with the knees being most commonly affected. Usually, the disease progresses slowly and results in:

- Pain in the affected joint
- Joint swelling and stiffness
- Fever
- Swelling of the feet, ankles and legs

Diagnosis

Diagnosis of fungal arthritis mainly relies on identifying the presence of a fungal infection and the type of the fungus. A joint aspiration will normally be carried out and, as can be seen from Figure 3.5, this is done by inserting a needle into the joint and withdrawing a sample of the synovial fluid. A culture of the joint fluid is then grown to identify the presence of microorganisms and to enable these to be identified.

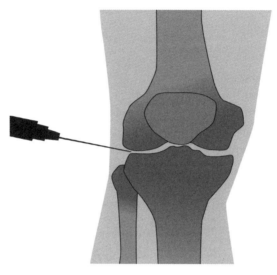

Figure 3.5 Joint aspiration

A synovial biopsy test may also be carried out under local anaesthetic and this essentially involves harvesting a small sample of tissue from within the joint for analysis. As certain microorganisms stimulate the body to produce antibodies when an active infection is present, a blood test may be taken to detect these, and X-rays of the affected joint(s) may also be able to pick up changes to the joint.

Treatment

Once the presence of a fungal infection of the joints has been identified, the main aim of treatment is to rid the body of the infection using antifungal drugs such as fluconazole, ketoconazole, itraconazole or amphotericin B. Where the condition is more advanced and the condition chronic, surgical removal of the infected tissue (known as debridement) may be necessary.

The prognosis for sufferers of fungal arthritis can depend largely on how long the condition remains untreated and on the underlying cause of the infection and the patient's general health. If fungal arthritis is allowed to develop untreated, it can cause long-term or permanent damage to the affected joint(s) and of course a weakened immune system or a disease such as cancer and the drugs used to treat it can vastly affect the patient's outcome.

Gout

Understanding the Condition

Gout is a condition which most people probably think of in relation to excess consumption of alcohol, and whilst this can indeed cause this particular form of arthritis, heavy drinkers are not the only ones who fall into the higher risk category. Those who are overweight or use certain types of medication, as well as people whose diets are high in particular types of food can also be more prone to attacks of gout. Before we look at why these things are relevant to the disease, however, let us first consider precisely what gout is and how it occurs.

Gout is a type of arthritis in which inflammation of the joints is caused by the build-up of uric acid and the formation of uric acid crystals in and around the joints, and it is often considered to be the most painful of all of the forms of the disease. Characterised by recurrent attacks during which the inflamed joint becomes hot, red, shiny, swollen and intensely painful and which typically last from a few days up to two weeks, the condition does not usually cause any permanent damage when the first few bouts are experienced. As can be seen from Figure 3.6, however, with repeated attacks, gout can damage the bone and the cartilage within the joint and lead to chronic arthritis. In addition to uric acid crystals forming within the joints, they can also develop just below the surface of the skin, appearing as firm, white lumps known as tophi. While often these do not create any particular problems in themselves, they can sometimes become inflamed and cause discomfort.

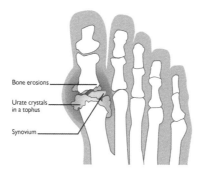

Figure 3.6 The effects of gout on a toe joint
Uric acid is a natural waste product which comes from the breakdown of purines and it is usually expelled from the body through the kidneys and into the urine. Purines, alongside being found in all of the cells of the body and forming part of the chemical structure of human and animal genes, are also present in the genes of plants and so exist at different levels of concentration in virtually all of the foods that we eat. If the amount of purines that we take into our bodies is reasonable and the body's systems work efficiently to metabolise them into uric acid and then remove them, then no problems are likely to develop. Where the intake of purines is high or the ability of the body to process uric acid is compromised in some way, however, then the acid builds up in the bloodstream and forms crystals in and around the joints.

Risk Factors for Developing the Condition
Some types of food contain very concentrated amounts of purines and so a diet which is high in these particular foodstuffs can increase the risk of gout, including:

- Liver
- Kidney
- Brains
- Sweetbreads
- Oily fish such as mackerel, sardines, herring and anchovies
- Mussels
- Meat extracts
- Yeast

High or moderately high levels of purines can also be found in:

- Bacon
- Beef
- Lamb
- Goose
- Duck
- Mutton
- Rabbit
- Turkey
- Chicken
- Veal
- Venison
- Pork
- Ham
- Tripe
- Salmon
- Cod
- Snapper
- Tuna
- Haibut
- Trout
- Crab
- Lobster
- Oysters
- Shellfish
- Cauliflower
- Mushrooms
- Spinach
- Peas
- Asparagus
- Kidney beans
- Lentils
- Lima beans
- Oatmeal

Despite the fact that all of these foodstuffs are known to contain very high, high or moderately high levels of purines, however, some research which has been carried out on tens of thousands of men and women has shown that purines which come from different sources have greater or lesser potential to increase the chances of suffering from gout. Purines from fish or meat, for example, are believed to increase the risk, while vegetables do not change it and dairy foods, which can also contain purines, are thought to lower the likelihood of suffering from the condition.

Purines and the uric acid which is produced when they are broken down are desirable in the body because they help to protect the blood vessels from damage, but as I have mentioned, the danger occurs when the levels become too high or the body cannot process the uric acid efficiently. Some of the factors which might cause the latter include:

- A genetic tendency for the kidneys to retain more uric acid than is normal

- Kidney disease which affects the ability of the organs to process uric acid as well as they should
- Blood disorders which cause the body to produce too many blood cells which, when broken down, produce more uric acid than the kidneys can cope with
- Medications such as diuretics which flush water from the body can increase levels of uric acid to such an extent that the kidneys cannot cope with them efficiently

In addition, high blood pressure, heart disease and diabetes are all associated with high levels of uric acid in the body and therefore increased risk of gout, although the reasons for this are not currently fully understood. As with other types of disease, where gout occurs as the result of an identified cause, it is generally described as secondary gout, but in most cases this form of arthritis is actually attributable to a combination of different factors and those who are prone to the disease can find that certain things trigger an attack, such as:

- A bruise or injury to a joint
- Undergoing surgery
- Having a tooth extracted
- Dehydration
- Illness
- Exhaustion
- Excessive eating
- Excessive consumption of alcohol

Although gout can affect the ankles, knees, hands, wrists and elbows, it is most commonly found in the lowest part of the body, in the big toe. In the vast majority of cases only a single joint is affected, but up to 10% of people experience pain and inflammation in more than one joint.

According to the UK Gout Society, men are five times more likely than women to suffer from this form of arthritis, which occurs most frequently in men between the ages of 40 and 60. In fact, gout is the most common form of inflammatory joint disease in men over 40. Although the condition can affect women and children, in both cases this would be a rare occurrence and, in the former, onset prior to menopause would be highly unusual.

Research has shown that gout does sometimes appear to run in families. In around 10% of cases there is a family history of the condition, although the reasons for this are not fully understood. As families very often follow similar eating and drinking patterns, both in terms of the types of foods and drinks that they consume as well as the quantities, this in itself may well account for the tendency for the condition to affect a number of members of the same family. As well as diet and being overweight, having high blood pressure also seems to set up a predisposition towards gout, but as this too is often linked with rich diets and the excess consumption of alcohol and sugar, the connection may again be a dietary one.

As I mentioned previously, attacks of gout can last anywhere from a few days to a couple of weeks (usually the latter), after which time the symptoms tend to disappear and the joints return to normal. While there are instances of people only ever experiencing a single attack during their lifetimes, usually there are repeated bouts which often occur for no obvious reason, although drinking too much alcohol or illness can act as triggers.

Diagnosis

A preliminary diagnosis of gout can usually be made based on the presentation of symptoms, an examination of the joints, the patient's family medical history and a description of lifestyle factors such as diet and alcohol consumption. Typically though, physicians will carry out blood tests to measure the levels of uric acid in the body. Although these tests cannot in themselves definitively confirm or refute a diagnosis of the condition, they can strongly support it. Part of the difficulty in relying solely on the results of these tests lies in the facts that levels of uric acid can not only be elevated as the result of other conditions such as diabetes and heart disease, but even during the course of an acute attack of gout the amount of acid in the blood can still show as normal.

The collection and microscopic examination of synovial fluid from the joint, while it can result in a conclusive diagnosis of gout, is not always a practical option where the condition affects small joints such as the big toe. Where it can be carried out, however, the uric acid crystals can be clearly seen under a microscope, leaving doctors in no doubt that their diagnosis was correct. X-rays, on the other hand, can provide evidence of chronic gout which has caused damage to the affected joint(s), but as such damage tends not to occur in the early years of the condition, they are rarely helpful during this time.

Treatment

Once a diagnosis of gout has been made, there are a number of medications that can be used to treat it. Non-steroidal anti-inflammatory drugs (NSAIDs) can be taken to alleviate pain and inflammation, although it is important to note that aspirin should be avoided unless prescribed by a doctor at a low dosage to protect against heart disease or similar conditions, as it can increase the levels of uric acid in the body.

A drug by the name of colchicine, meanwhile, acts to inhibit the migration of white blood cells into the inflamed area. White blood cells move in to try and overwhelm uric acid crystals in the joints, but when they do so, lactic acid and enzymes which cause inflammation are released and lead to pain and swelling. By stopping this migration, colchicine can help to alleviate the pain and swelling of gout, but it does have certain contraindications for some patients, as well as being responsible for a number of unpleasant side effects. Should these contraindications or side effects make it impossible to take colchicine or should the condition not respond favourably to this drug or to NSAIDs, then a steroid injection may be given directly into the joint or steroid tablets prescribed to be taken orally for a few days.

Although the medications mentioned so far are aimed at relieving the symptoms of gout, what they cannot do is affect the levels of uric acid in the blood. If these are shown by blood tests to be high, therefore, or if attacks of gout become more frequent, then it may be necessary to prescribe one of a different group of drugs to reduce the levels. Medications such as allopurinol, sold under the brand name of Zyloprim, are normally taken indefinitely unless they result in side effects, as it can take as long as two years for the body to be completely cleared of uric acid crystals. These drugs also need to be taken on a regular and uninterrupted basis, as any interruptions to dosages can result in the triggering of acute attacks of gout. Alongside taking medications which are designed to lower uric acid levels, however, it is also important for patients to make appropriate changes to their diets and levels of alcohol consumption and, if necessary, to lose any excess weight so that any future build-up of acid and the associated formation of crystals in the joints is avoided.

Although earlier bouts of gout are unlikely to cause any harm to the joints, as I have said, repeated attacks can lead to permanent damage to the cartilage and bone and to chronic arthritis, making early treatment and control of the disease important. As well as taking prescription medications to manage the condition, ice packs can be used to help soothe the affected joint and during painful episodes protecting the joint such as by using a cage to take the weight of bedclothes can be helpful. Sufferers of gout should also be sure to drink plenty of water, as this helps to stop the uric acid from crystallising in the joints. Alcohol, and particularly beer, sugary soft drinks and large quantities of tea and coffee, however, should be avoided.

Although gout does not normally lead to any further problems, if uric acid crystals collect in the urinary tract, then kidney stones can be the result, and if they collect in the tissue of the kidneys then this can cause damage to the kidneys themselves. In the vast majority of cases, however, the prognosis for gout sufferers is good, provided that patients take prescribed medications as directed and follow the recommended lifestyle changes carefully. If these things are done, then there is every likelihood that the levels of uric acid in the body can be sufficiently reduced that the symptoms disappear altogether.

Juvenile Idiopathic Arthritis

The terminology in relation to arthritis which affects children and adolescents is currently very confusing and so, before I look at how youngsters are affected by the disease, it is probably worthwhile just making a few distinctions.

First of all, what I have referred to in the heading above as 'juvenile idiopathic arthritis' or JIA was, and sometimes still is known as juvenile rheumatoid arthritis. The reason for evolving to the use of JIA is because the term 'juvenile rheumatoid arthritis' tends to suggest a 'junior' version of adult rheumatoid arthritis, when in fact the two conditions are very different. JIA is also sometimes referred to as juvenile chronic arthritis, but this term is also confusing because there are forms of childhood arthritis other than JIA which are chronic but which are not encompassed by the term JIA. Juvenile ankylosing spondylitis and juvenile psoriatic arthritis, for example, are chronic forms of arthritis which affect youngsters, but they are not included in the definition of JIA.

The word 'idiopathic' is used to refer to diseases or conditions for which the cause is unknown and so, for the sake of clarity, I will use the term JIA to mean inflammation of the joint which has no defined cause and which begins before the age of 16. I will discuss the different types of JIA in this section, before considering other types of childhood arthritis under the following heading of 'Juvenile Spondyloarthritis'.

It is estimated that around 12,000 children in the UK and around 300,000 in the USA are affected by some form of arthritis and many of these cases fall into the category of JIA. In some cases symptoms last for only a few weeks or months and never return, whilst in others they continue well into adulthood and, in rare cases, sometimes even throughout the individual's lifetime. As the term 'idiopathic' suggests, there is no clear cause for the condition, but the presence of certain antibodies which attack the body's tissues and organs (known as autoantibodies) does suggest that JIA is an autoimmune disease.

JIA is normally categorised into one of three main types – pauciarticular, polyarticular and systemic – and although the severity of cases can vary considerably within each category, generally it is considered that the order in which the different types have been listed here is from least to most severe. To follow, you will find a description of each.

Pauciarticular JIA

Pauciarticular JIA, which is sometimes also referred to as oligoarticular JIA, is the most common and generally the mildest form of the condition and is believed to account for around 50% of all cases. The terms 'pauciarticular' and 'oligoarticular' both mean 'few joints' and, in this type of JIA, four or fewer joints are affected. Typically, symptoms are experienced in particular joints on one side of the body only and although the condition can affect the spine, wrists or the smaller joints in the fingers or toes, usually it is in the larger weight-bearing joints such as the knees, ankles and elbows that pain and swelling tend to occur.

Within the category of pauciarticular JIA, there are two distinct groups of children who are affected. The first is girls under the age of 7, who in one-third of cases not only experience joint pain and inflammation, but also a type of inflammation of the eye which is known as iridocyclitis or uveitis and which affects the front part of the eye between the cornea (the clear window at the front of the eye) and the lens. Typically, the condition causes pain, soreness and redness of the eye, sensitivity to light and blurred vision. Usually it is only experienced in one eye at a time but may alternate between eyes with repeated attacks. If left untreated, the inflammation can cause permanent damage in one of several ways:

- By causing the lens and the iris to stick together
- By causing clouding of the lens (cataract) and blurred vision
- By causing the pressure in the eye to increase, which can in turn lead to glaucoma, a condition in which the nerve in the eye is damaged and in which there is the potential for permanent loss of vision

Sufferers of pauciarticular arthritis who fall into this group and who develop symptoms of iridocyclitis should be taken to see an ophthalmologist within 24 hours in order for the diagnosis to be confirmed and the treatment started. Better still, however, girls under seven with this form of arthritis should be subjected to an anti-nuclear antibody (ANA) test at the time of diagnosis in order to determine whether there is a greater risk of iridocyclitis, and then the situation monitored thereafter.

The second group to be affected by pauciarticular JIA includes boys over the age of eight and, in this case, it is the sacroiliac joints in the lower part of the spine as depicted in Figure 3.7, the hips, knees and ankles which become inflamed. Tendons and the points at which these and ligaments attach to bones also suffer from inflammation and the child may additionally develop chronic irido-cyclitis. In some children, and particularly those who have the *HLA-B27* gene, this type of JIA may indicate the presence of or the predisposition towards one of the forms of spondyloarthritis discussed in the following section.

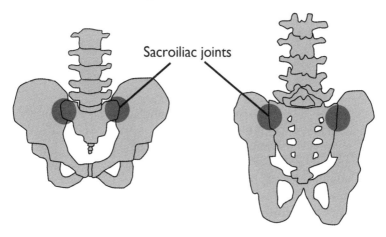

Sacroiliac joints

Anterior (front) view   Posterior (rear) view

Figure 3.7 The sacroiliac joints

Although most cases of pauciarticular JIA do not lead to long-term joint problems, if the condition is chronic it can result in damage to the cartilage, enlargement of the joint, the shortening or length-ening of a limb or digit and/or limited range of motion in a joint. In some cases, however, it is the risk of chronic damage to the eyes which is greater than that to the joints.

Polyarticular JIA
Polyarticular JIA is a form of juvenile arthritis which affects five or more joints in the body and it is believed to account for 30–40% of cases of JIA. In this case, the onset may occur at any age in boys or

girls, but the condition tends to affect more girls than boys. Symptoms tend to be more severe than in pauciarticular JIA and when polyarticular JIA affects teenagers the disease frequently manifests itself in similar ways to adult-onset rheumatoid arthritis.

In some ways, the characteristics of polyarticular JIA are completely opposite to those of the pauciarticular form. While the latter generally only affects a joint on one side of the body, the former tends to present symmetrically. In addition, it is typically the smaller joints in the fingers and hands which are impacted by polyarticular JIA, although in some cases the hips, knees and ankles, as well as the neck or jaw, may be affected. Joint pain and inflammation may also be accompanied by:

- Tiredness
- Low-grade fever
- Nodules on parts of the body which are subject to pressure, such as the elbows or parts of the feet
- Stiffness in the neck and difficulty in turning the head
- Pain and discomfort in the jaw when chewing (due to retarded growth in the jaw)
- Anaemia
- Iridocyclitis (particularly in girls under seven)

Although not particularly common, some children may also experience inflammation of the internal organs and tests for rheumatoid factor (RF) may indicate the presence of the autoantibody which usually shows up in cases of adult-onset rheumatoid arthritis.

Systemic JIA

The most serious of all of the types of JIA is systemic JIA, formerly called Still's disease. Responsible for around 10–15% of the reported cases of JIA, it not only affects any number of the joints in the body, but the entire bodily system and in some cases the organs.

Systemic JIA affects boys and girls equally and it often begins with symptoms which are similar to those of infection. Fever, lethargy, swollen glands and rashes are common in the early stages, but pain and inflammation in the joints and muscles, and sometimes in the internal organs, are also typical. Body temperatures can reach 103 degrees or higher and the patient may experience fevers on a daily basis for weeks or months. A rash of pale or dark pink spots may appear on the chest, thighs or other parts of the body independently or in conjunction with spells of fever and often it will come and go over the course of many days. Joint pain too may accompany the fever, but in some cases does not appear until weeks or months later. In some cases the symptoms which are not directly related to the joints disappear completely within the first few months of the illness, with those which are joint-related becoming a much longer-term problem. Eventually, many of the joints in the body can become affected by pain, swelling and stiffness.

For some sufferers of systemic JIA, additional problems occur in the form of inflammation of the lining of the heart (pericarditis) or lungs (pleurisy), as well as with anaemia. High numbers of white blood cells (which attack bacteria and infections) may also be evident when blood tests are carried out and if these tests also show elevated platelet levels there can be an increase in the risk of a blood clot forming. The condition can, in addition, lead to enlarged lymph nodes, liver or spleen and so monitoring via regular and frequent blood tests is important during the early stages of the disease. Problems with the eyes, which are quite common in pauciarticular and polyarticular arthritis, however, are much less common with this form of the condition.

Around 50% of the children who suffer from systemic JIA are free from symptoms within one year of the onset of the condition, but the illness can sometimes return without warning or in the wake of certain types of viral infection such as chicken pox. However, with ongoing treatment for both systemic and joint symptoms, which may be required for a period of months or years, there is a great deal that can be done to control the disease and minimise the chances of any long-term damage.

In terms of the effects of JIA on the joints of youngsters, as can be seen from Figure 3.8, the synovial membrane which makes up the joint capsule thickens and becomes filled with inflammatory cells, and the amount of synovial fluid within the capsule increases, causing swelling, pain and restrictions to movement which tend to be worse first thing in the morning or after periods of inactivity. If these symptoms remain untreated, then this can eventually lead to erosion of the cartilage and bone, which then tries to repair itself and produces bony overgrowths.

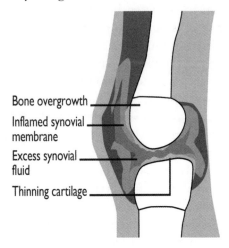

Bone overgrowth
Inflamed synovial membrane
Excess synovial fluid
Thinning cartilage

Figure 3.8 Joint affected by JIA

As is common with people of any age who suffer from arthritis, children also try to reduce the amount of pain that they experience by keeping the affected joint in a half-bent position. This, however, not only tends to increase the feeling of stiffness, but also to cause the muscles and soft tissues around the joint to lose strength and waste away, making normal movement even more difficult.

Diagnosis

Regardless of which type of JIA a child is diagnosed with, the nature and severity of symptoms can vary greatly from one to another, but in each case an early and accurate diagnosis is important if long-term damage to eyes, joints or organs is to be avoided. Normally, diagnosis of the particular type of arthritis is made when there has been persistent pain and swelling in the joints for six weeks or more, but even then there is no single test which can detect JIA. After taking the child's full medical history and carrying out a physical examination, doctors will normally then do a number of tests which are designed both to confirm a suspected diagnosis of JIA as well as to rule out other possible illnesses, especially other forms of arthritis which might have similar symptoms. These might include, for example, tests to identify the presence of the *HLA-B27* gene, erythrocyte sedimentation rate (ESR), antinuclear antibody (ANA) and blood count tests. In addition, samples of fluid or tissue may be taken from the affected joints to check for infection or inflammation and X-rays and scans may be carried out to identify whether there is any evidence of infection, tumour or fracture.

Treatment

Once a definitive diagnosis has been reached, the aim of treatment is not only to alleviate the pain and swelling in the joints and prevent any long-term damage or loss of mobility, but also to ensure that the vital internal organs and the eyes are protected. In addition to taking what might be a number of different medications to control symptoms, a multidisciplinary treatment regime will normally encompass physical therapies and exercise programmes, as well as recommendations for the wearing of special equipment such as splints to hold the joints in the correct position and relieve pain, and any necessary changes to diet and lifestyle. Because the wide range of treatments involves a number of different specialists often much more beneficial results are achieved from working with a pain management facility which can provide a co-ordinated treatment plan.

In terms of the drugs which are used to treat JIA, these will of course depend on the type of the condition and the severity of the symptoms. In rare cases, aspirin may be prescribed in fairly high doses to control pain, swelling and fever, but more often non-steroidal anti-inflammatory drugs such as ibuprofen and naproxen are recommended. Slow-acting anti-rheumatic drugs (SAARDs) and disease-modifying anti-rheumatic drugs (DMARDs), meanwhile, may be taken to alter the progress of the disease and reduce the risk of damage to cartilage and bone. As the latter are powerful medications which, like all drugs, can cause side effects, frequent monitoring is necessary to ensure that they are safe and appropriate for the child to continue taking.

Another type of drug which is commonly prescribed in moderate to severe cases of JIA is one of the group of immunosuppressants. These medications are designed to inhibit the activity of the immune system, so helping to reduce inflammation in addition to slowing down the thickening of the synovial membrane that surrounds the joints. Methotrexate, which is also used to treat certain types of cancer as well as adult-onset rheumatoid arthritis, is one of the more popular immunosuppressants used for JIA, but because the dosages prescribed for children with this condition are much lower than those used for cancer patients, side effects are much less significant and less frequent. While some immunosuppressant drugs are given orally, either in liquid or pill form, others may be administered by injection.

A newer group of drugs known as biologic agents, which were developed for the treatment of rheumatoid arthritis, are also used in some cases of JIA. These medications, such as etanercept and infliximab, are genetically-engineered drugs which work by interfering with the biologic substances in the body that cause or worsen inflammation, and they can specifically affect some of the abnormalities of the immune system which result in joint inflammation. Glucocorticoids, a class of steroid hormones whose anti-inflammatory properties are extremely powerful, meanwhile, may be prescribed at the lowest possible dose and for the shortest possible amount of time in severe cases of JIA and those in which other medications have failed to alleviate inflammation. However, as these drugs are known for producing a variety of side effects extreme care needs to be taken in terms of monitoring, and discontinuance of the medication should only be done gradually and under proper medical supervision. Children who are taking glucocorticoids are also advised to wear a medical alert bracelet or necklace to alert medical personnel to this fact in the event of accident or emergency surgery.

As I mentioned earlier, alongside the taking of pharmaceutical drugs, physical therapies and exercise play an extremely important role in the treatment of JIA. Not only do these help to keep joints mobile and reduce the chances of disability, but they also build up muscle and ensure good levels of general fitness and stamina. For children in particular, avoiding the physical limitations that can potentially develop with juvenile arthritis is vital if they are going to be able to enjoy a normal childhood and participate in activities with friends and family. With the help of a trained physical therapist, children can learn which exercises are most beneficial for their particular symptoms and how to perform these exercises properly at home. Techniques such as muscle relaxation, controlled breathing and guided imagery can also be extremely useful in terms of managing and controlling pain.

While a good, nutritious diet is, of course, important for all children, those with JIA need to take particular care. While the pain and other symptoms that they experience can often lead to suppressed appetites and so to weight loss and poor growth, the side effects of some medications coupled with the inability or unwillingness to take part in physical activities can lead to excessive weight gain. Ensuring that children receive the appropriate intake of calories and food which has high nutritional content therefore is vital if they are going to be properly equipped to deal with the increased demands that the disease places on their bodies. As carrying excess weight puts additional stress on the knees, hips and ankles in particular, sticking to a healthy, balanced diet and taking the appropriate amount of exercise not only ensures better overall health, but also that no further and unnecessary damage to the joints is sustained.

Although surgery is rarely necessary in cases of JIA, it may sometimes be recommended in cases where permanently tightened muscles, tendons and ligaments are causing severe pain or when joints have been damaged. Because the child may still be growing, typically joint replacement surgery will be delayed until such time as the growing process is almost or fully complete.

One aspect of treatment that I have not yet touched on but which is particularly important in the case of juvenile arthritis is education. Not only does it help children themselves to understand their condition, how best to manage their symptoms and what changes might be beneficial to their lifestyles, but it is also immensely reassuring for parents too. From the more practical aspects of the illness such as ensuring a healthy diet and communicating problems and restrictions to schools, to learning how to maintain a routine and a home environment which is as normal as possible, parents can do much to contribute to their child's immediate and long-term recovery and prospects and so ensure that they are able to grow up as active and productive members of society.

Juvenile Spondyloarthritis

Understanding the Condition
Although the term 'spondylo' actually means 'of the spine', spondyloarthritis (sometimes referred to as spondyloarthropathy) refers to a group of arthritic conditions which typically involve the joints in the spine, as well as peripheral joints such as the pelvis, hips, knees and ankles. In addition, there tends to be inflammation in the areas where ligaments and tendons attach to bone (known as entheses) and inflammation of the skin, eyes and intestines. In children under the age of 16, the family of conditions is known as juvenile spondyloarthritis and includes:

- Juvenile ankylosing spondylitis
- Psoriatic arthritis
- Reactive arthritis
- A type of arthritis which is associated with inflammatory bowel disease
- Undifferentiated spondyloarthropathy, in which the symptoms cannot be classified as a specific rheumatic disorder

These conditions may continue into or even throughout the adult life of the sufferer, but the course of the disease varies greatly from one child to another and in some cases it may last for only a matter of months and then go into complete remission.

Although the types of arthritis which are grouped under the heading of juvenile spondyloarthritis might not at first seem to bear much in common, in fact they do share certain features in that they all tend to:

- Involve the spine, and especially the sacroiliac joints at the junction of the spine and the pelvis
- Only affect a joint on one side of the body rather than symmetrical joints
- Affect mainly large joints
- Involve the entheses
- Cause inflammation of the eyes
- Appear in people who have the *HLA-B27* gene

Another thing that children who are diagnosed with juvenile spondyloarthritis have in common is that they will be classed as 'seronegative', which basically means that blood tests for rheumatoid factor will show a negative result. Rheumatoid factor is an antibody which is not normally found in the blood of the majority of the population (only 1–2% of healthy people test positive) but which is found in upwards of 80% of people who have rheumatoid arthritis, as well as in some of those who suffer from certain other conditions such as Sjögren's syndrome and scleroderma.

In the case of reactive and psoriatic arthritis, the symptoms in children present in much the same ways as in adults and you can read more about each of these conditions under the appropriate headings. With juvenile ankylosing spondylitis, however, it is not uncommon for symptoms in the spine to appear much later than those in other joints of the body, and it can even be years before any involvement with the back becomes evident. In these cases, the child is typically diagnosed with enthesitis-related arthritis (i.e. the type of arthritis which causes inflammation of the sites where the ligaments and tendons attach to the bones) in the first instance, with the diagnosis being changed as full-blown juvenile ankylosing spondylitis develops, something which is estimated to happen in as many as 50% of cases.

Enthesitis-related arthritis, or ERA for short, tends to affect the larger weight-bearing joints in the lower part of the body, and particularly the hips and knees. Pain and tenderness due to inflammation of the entheses is also common, especially in the sites above and below the kneecap, at the back of the heel and underneath it, and in the ball of the foot. In some cases it can also affect the shoulders, although elbows and wrists are rarely involved.

Iridocyclitis also tends to occur in around 50% of cases, but although in some other forms of juvenile arthritis this is not always accompanied by redness or pain in the eyes, in ERA it generally is.

The type of arthritis associated with inflammatory bowel disease, on the other hand, is one which can occur as a manifestation of Crohn's disease or ulcerative colitis. These cases tend to involve the joints in the arms or legs and may also affect the joints in the spine, particularly in children who have the *HLA-B27* **gene.**

Undifferentiated spondyloarthritis, as the name suggests, is the diagnosis which is given if the criteria for the other conditions are not specifically met. Sometimes, however, symptoms do become more well-defined over time, in which case the diagnosis may be changed to one of juvenile ankylosing spondylitis or one of the other related diseases which fall under the heading of juvenile spondyloarthritis.

Although the exact cause of juvenile spondyloarthritis is not known, the facts that so many sufferers have the *HLA-B27* gene and that the illnesses which fall within this group often run in families do tend to suggest that hereditary factors play an important role. As has been described under the earlier headings, as there is no single test which can diagnose any of the specific diseases which fall into the group of juvenile spondyloarthropathies, a variety of tests may be carried out to rule in or out the various forms of arthritis (as well as other medical conditions which present with similar symptoms, such as fibromyalgia) and if there is no evidence of ankylosing spondylitis, psoriasis, Crohn's disease or ulcerative colitis and nothing to suggest a previous infection in the body, the patient will normally be diagnosed with undifferentiated spondyloarthritis.

Treatment

In terms of treatments for juvenile spondyloarthritis, non-steroidal anti-inflammatory drugs (NSAIDs) such as ibuprofen are often the first line of attack. Corticosteroid injections directly into the joint space, however, can also help to significantly reduce inflammation, with the effects of a single injection sometimes lasting for as long as six months. Disease-modifying anti-rheumatic drugs (DMARDs) have also been found to be helpful in some cases, as have biologic agents, but if either of these types of drugs are prescribed, there will normally be regular monitoring of the child for side effects.

As with all types of adult-onset or juvenile arthritis, physical therapy and exercise are extremely important elements of treatment in cases of juvenile spondyloarthritis. The lives of children can be particularly badly affected in a physical, emotional, psychological and developmental sense if their condition places enormous restrictions on them, and so improving and maintaining strength and flexibility is vital to enable them to take part in normal everyday activities and those with their peers. A trained and qualified physical therapist will be able to recommend exercises and physical activities which are appropriate and safe for the child to carry out and, as part of a multidisciplinary treatment programme, specialists can also advise on equipment such as splints or special shoes or shoe inserts which can be used to minimise pain and allow the individual to maintain as normal a lifestyle as possible.

As there is currently no cure for juvenile spondyloarthritis and there is the potential for the condition to carry on throughout the sufferer's life, learning as much as possible about the disease itself and how best to cope with it is essential if a good quality of life is to be preserved. Research has shown time and time again that those who approach illness with a positive frame of mind, who accept their condition and who are prepared to incorporate the necessary lifestyle changes into their lives have a much better prognosis than those who do not. For children who are already undergoing many physical and emotional changes in the process of growing up, being diagnosed with a chronic condition can be extremely challenging, but at the same time youngsters are often more accepting of lifestyle changes if they are guided appropriately.

Parents too need to educate themselves about their child's condition and be actively involved in ensuring that he or she carries out the recommended physical activities. They also have an important role to play in liaising with teachers so that any special needs that the child might have are catered to and that if certain activities are to be avoided, such as high-impact sports, the school is aware of these.

Of course, for any parent, watching their child in pain can be an extremely distressing experience and there can be a tendency to change routines or make exceptions for a youngster who is clearly in some discomfort. Some children, for example, may try to avoid school because of their symptoms, which can clearly have serious adverse effects in later life if it happens regularly. Encouraging them to attend, as well as keeping a sense of normality in terms of all other aspects of daily life, therefore, is essential for their normal development, even though it may feel cruel at the time.

Polymyalgia Rheumatica

Understanding the Condition

Although most of the forms of arthritis that we have looked at so far affect the workings of the joints which are found inside the joint capsule, such as the ends of the bones and the cartilage, polymyalgia rheumatica, or PMR as it is commonly known, is a type of the disease which involves the muscles that surround and control the joints. In fact, the name of the condition comes from the Greek words 'poly' meaning many, 'myos' meaning muscles and 'algos' meaning pain.

According to Arthritis Research UK, PMR affects around 1 in every 2,000 people. The disease, however, does not usually start until after the age of 50, and in fact the average age of onset is around 70. Between two and three times more women are affected than men and some studies have shown that white people are at greater risk, and particularly those from the Scandinavian countries. Interestingly, the rate of prevalence of PMR is also reported to be above average in the east and south-east of England and below average in the north and north-west, which may suggest that there are environmental factors at play in the onset of the disease.

The symptoms of PMR are caused by inflammation of the muscles. Although the cause of the condition is currently unknown, some believe PMR to be an autoimmune disease in which the body's immune system attacks healthy tissues. As can be seen from Figure 3.9, most often it is the muscles surrounding the shoulder and hip joints which are affected, but often there is referred pain from these areas into the upper arms, buttocks and thighs.

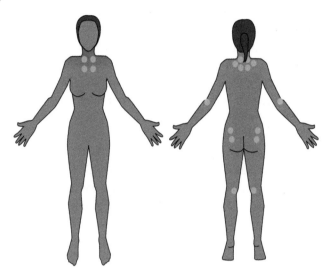

Figure 3.9 Areas of the body most commonly affected by PMR

The severe and widespread stiffness, pain, aching and tenderness which is associated with PMR typically feels worse in the mornings or after prolonged periods of inactivity and can make everyday tasks such as getting out of bed, dressing and negotiating stairs particularly difficult. Where the shoulders are affected, raising the arm above shoulder height, for instance to comb the hair, can present enormous difficulties, but symptoms generally ease as the day goes on. Although not always the case, inflammation of some of the soft tissues, such as the tendons, can also accompany the pain and stiffness, as can swelling of the hands, feet and other joints. In addition, there may also be other more general symptoms, including:

- Fever
- Depression
- Fatigue

- Night sweats
- Loss of appetite
- Weight loss

Although not always the case, the symptoms of PMR tend to develop fairly rapidly, usually over the course of a few days or weeks and sometimes even as quickly as overnight, a fact which often leads people to seek prompt diagnosis and treatment. In cases where the development of the condition is more gradual, however, it can be tempting for the sufferer to put the symptoms down to the aches and pains of old age at first and to put up with them until they become unbearable.

Diagnosis

As there is no single diagnostic test for PMR, diagnosis of the condition normally relies on the patient history, a description of current symptoms, a physical examination and a series of blood tests. If erythrocyte sedimentation rate (ESR) and C-reactive protein (CRP) tests show high levels of inflammation in the body, these can give clues as to the presence of PMR when considered alongside other symptoms which are typical of the condition. In addition, a test to check the level of red blood cells can detect anaemia, which is also quite common in cases of PMR, but if doubt still remains as to the cause of the symptoms, doctors may call for other tests to be carried out in order to rule out other illnesses.

Treatment

Although standard pain-relieving medications and anti-inflammatory drugs are often quite effective for some forms of arthritis, they tend not to be so in cases of PMR and so treatment to relieve inflammation tends to rely on the more powerful corticosteroids. These drugs normally bring about an improvement in symptoms within just a few days, but as they are not a cure for the condition and relapses can occur, they usually need to be taken over the course of two years or more. Because corticosteroids can cause side effects, however, including an increased risk of osteoporosis (thinning of the bone), doctors will normally try to reduce dosages as soon as symptoms appear to be under control. If doing so causes symptoms to return or if there are repeated relapses, immunosuppressants may also be prescribed to be taken in tandem with decreased doses of steroids. If long-term use of steroids is necessary, other medications may additionally be recommended to reduce the risk of osteoporosis.

Monitoring of patients who are being treated for PMR is an important part of the process as even low doses of corticosteroids can increase the risk of osteoporosis as well as a number of other unwanted side effects, of which weight gain and raised blood sugar levels are just two. As part of a multidisciplinary approach to treatment, specialists can advise on the right types of exercise to help maintain bone strength, as well as on changes to diet and nutrition which are aimed at improving calcium absorption and keeping weight under control. Drinking a pint of milk each day and eating calcium-rich foods, as well as increasing the intake of foods containing Vitamin D (which helps the body to absorb calcium) or taking Vitamin D supplements, for example, can all help to keep osteoporosis at bay, as can avoiding excessive amounts of alcohol and smoking.

Giant Cell Arteritis or Temporal Arteritis

Despite the fact that the prognosis for PMR is normally very good and that the condition responds very well to treatment, something which sufferers (as well as those who care for them) should be aware of is the link between this disease and another condition known as giant cell arteritis or temporal arteritis which needs prompt medical attention. Giant cell arteritis is a condition in which the arteries of the skull become painfully inflamed and it can cause damage to the arteries in the eyes. The symptoms typically present as:

- Severe headaches and pains in the muscles of the head
- Pain or swelling in the scalp
- Jaw pain
- Tenderness around the temple area
- Blurred or double vision, or even the loss of vision

It is estimated that around 20% of people with PMR will also suffer from giant cell arteritis and that 40–60% of sufferers of the latter will also have symptoms of PMR. The two conditions often appear at the same time, which has led some experts to question whether they might not even be symptoms of a single medical condition which has not yet been identified.

Where giant cell arteritis is suspected typically a biopsy of a small piece of artery will be taken from the scalp for analysis and, if the diagnosis is confirmed, then a higher dose of corticosteroids will be prescribed to treat both this condition and PMR. If giant cell arteritis is diagnosed and treated before there is any loss of vision, then the prognosis is normally good and patients do not suffer any serious after-effects. If there is a delay in diagnosis and treatment, however, it is likely that any loss of vision will be permanent.

Polymyositis and Dermatomyositis

Understanding the Condition

The term 'myositis' literally means 'inflammation of the muscles' and both polymyositis and dermatomyositis are conditions in which the muscles undergo degenerative changes which cause them to become progressively weaker, even to the point of severe disability. While in polymyositis many muscles in the body are affected ('poly' comes from the Greek word for 'many'), in dermatomyositis there is also a component which affects the skin.

Polymyositis and dermatomyositis are rare conditions which are thought to affect no more than 5–10 people in every 100,000. Although the vast majority of these are adults, an estimated two to three cases of juvenile dermatomyositis are also reported each year per every one million people. In adults, the cases affecting women outnumber those affecting men by 2:1, but the rate of incidence does not seem to be any higher or lower in different races. Those between the ages of 50 and 60 seem to be more prone to polymyositis, while the incidence of dermatomyositis peaks between 45 and 65.

Polymyositis and dermatomyositis are both believed to be auto-immune disorders and, although there is no evidence that they are passed on through families, some think that a hereditary abnormality in the immune system may set up a predisposition to the conditions in certain people. In most cases, it is the larger muscles in the hips, shoulders and thighs which are first affected and typically the effects are felt on both sides of the body. Symptoms of muscle weakness normally appear gradually over the course of weeks or months but become progressively worse as time goes on.

In polymyositis, the sufferer may experience:

- Difficulties in walking, rising from a chair, climbing stairs or lifting objects, as well as raising the arms, for example to comb the hair. Where the neck muscles are affected, there may also be difficulties in raising the head, such as from a pillow
- Muscle weakness which varies from week to week and month to month
- Muscle pain and cramps
- Swelling and the build-up of fluid in the joints
- Fatigue
- Difficulties in swallowing (dysphagia) due to weakness in the muscles of the throat
- Inflammation which causes muscles to feel tender to the touch
- General feeling of being unwell
- Weight loss
- Night sweats
- Raynaud's phenomenon, in which the blood vessels in the hands and/or feet become constricted

Several things are quite notable about polymyositis. First of all, unlike in dermatomyositis, only about one-third of patients suffer from any pain as a result of the condition. In addition, although the effects of polymyositis can be extremely evident in the larger muscles of the body, the smaller muscles, such as in the hands, suffer no ill-effects until very much later in the disease. This means that tasks such as writing or buttoning a shirt, which require great dexterity, usually remain completely unaffected throughout most of the course of the illness. Also, many believe that polymyositis is likely to progress more slowly than dermatomyositis.

Another thing which is quite significant about polymyositis is that it often goes hand-in-hand with one of the other autoimmune diseases such as systemic lupus erythematosus, Sjögren's syndrome, rheumatoid arthritis or scleroderma. In fact, in a disease whose symptoms can be so diverse and in which levels of severity can vary so greatly, it is often this association with one of these other conditions that gives doctors clues in terms of diagnosis.

Dermatomyositis, although it presents in many of the same ways as polymyositis, also has additional symptoms which can sometimes resemble those of scleroderma (discussed later on in this chapter). These symptoms might include:

- Muscle pain and tenderness which appears during the early stages of the disease
- A skin rash which is often patchy and a blue-purple colour on the upper eyelids and red or pink on the face, neck, hands, shoulders and trunk. Where changes to the skin appear over the joints, such as the knuckles, elbows and knees, the rash may be scaly, slightly raised and purple-red in colour. Rashes may become worse if the sufferer is exposed to direct sunlight
- White lumps under the surface of the skin where calcium deposits have collected (calcinosis)
- In juvenile dermatomyositis, calcium deposits within the muscles which can lead to permanently bent joints
- Degeneration of the blood vessels (vasculitis)
- Thickening of the base and sides of the fingernails
- Rough or cracked skin on the sides and fronts of the fingers
- Fever
- Joint pain
- Gastrointestinal infections and ulcers
- Inflammation of the lung tissues

Dermatomyositis is seen much more commonly in children than polymyositis and the disease typically progresses rapidly and is much more severe. In some cases where symptoms appear suddenly and the patient experiences difficulties in breathing or swallowing, it may even be necessary for them to be admitted to hospital urgently until the condition has been stabilised.

Diagnosis

The characteristic skin rash which appears as one of the key symptoms of dermatomyositis, as well as a typical pattern of muscle weakness, should in many ways make this form of the condition quite recognisable. One of the difficulties with diagnosis, however, lies in the fact that the disease is so rare, particularly in children, making it hard for physicians who have no experience of the condition to identify it. In polymyositis, meanwhile, the symptoms may be confused with late-onset muscular dystrophy or certain other conditions which cause muscle weakness and pain. While tests to check the erythrocyte sedimentation rate (ESR) and the levels of creatine phosphokinase (an enzyme which leaks out of damaged muscles) might, therefore, help to rule out other conditions, they cannot conclusively confirm a diagnosis of either of these diseases and so are likely to be carried out in conjunction with a muscle biopsy.

A muscle biopsy involves taking a small sample of muscle to check for chronic inflammation, as well as the muscle degeneration and regeneration which is typical of polymyositis and dermatomyositis. Ideally, the sample should be taken from a muscle which, on clinical examination, shows weakness, and in which inflammation has been detected by an MRI scan. Additionally, an electromyography (EMG) test, which is designed to detect and record electrical discharges from nerve endings, should also have shown an abnormal pattern of electrical activity. Should microscopic examination of the sample indicate abnormal clumps of proteins inside the muscle cells, a definitive diagnosis of polymyositis or dermatomyositis can be given.

Although there is no evidence to suggest an association between juvenile dermatomyositis and the development of cancer, in rare cases of adult polymyositis and dermatomyositis there does appear to be a link. In addition to carrying out tests to diagnose the arthritic condition, therefore, doctors may also arrange for additional X-rays or scans to check that there are no tumours present.

Treatment

Once the diagnosis of polymyositis or dermatomyositis has been confirmed, a range of different drug therapies can be prescribed to treat the condition. Relatively high doses of corticosteroids are normally used as the first line of attack and these generally bring about a rapid reduction in inflammation. However, as these drugs do have a number of potential side effects, including an increased risk of osteoporosis, dosages are reduced as quickly as possible. In addition, although the inflammation may quickly die down, the muscles themselves do take a number of weeks or even months to repair themselves and so strength is normally only regained gradually. During the period when the inflammation is still subsiding, patients are usually advised to curtail some of their normal activities in order to prevent more damage from occurring.

In cases where corticosteroids are largely ineffective, where the patient relies on moderate to high dosages of the drug, where complications arise with the use of the medication or symptoms flare up when the dosage is reduced, then immunosuppressants such as methotrexate, cyclosporine or intravenous immunoglobulin can be used to suppress the immune system and so reduce inflammation. As these drugs can also have side effects, blood tests will normally be carried out at regular intervals during the course of treatment, both as a precautionary measure and to ensure that the treatment is working.

Even in more severe cases of polymyositis and dermatomyositis, drug treatments are normally very effective, although some patients do continue to experience some muscle weakness and others require ongoing treatment to keep the condition under control. Those people in whom the muscles used for breathing and swallowing are affected may require medical assistance to help them breathe or eat in addition to treatments to reduce muscle inflammation.

Although, as I have mentioned, curtailing some normal activities may be advisable when the disease is active, because polymyositis and dermatomyositis are conditions which can cause the muscles to atrophy or waste, it is important to begin exercising as soon as the disease starts to settle. A trained and qualified physiotherapist will be able to recommend appropriate exercises which are designed to restore muscle strength and improve stamina and these will normally be carried out under supervision in the first instance and then continued by the patient at home. Because of the particular risk of children's joints becoming permanently bent when calcium deposits invade the damaged muscles, the physiotherapy exercises which are recommended are likely to be quite vigorous, but it is important that these be carried out if long-term disability is to be avoided.

The prognosis for sufferers of polymyositis or dermatomyositis can be highly variable and much will depend on the extent of any involvement of the muscles of the heart or lungs and on whether cancer develops as a result of the condition. Both diseases are normally active in adults and children for a period of two to three years, unless there are heart or lung complications, in which case this period may be extended. Within five years, however, an estimated 50% of sufferers go into long-term or even permanent remission and in adults there is a 75% survival rate within this time span. In children the rate is even higher.

The number of people who make a full and complete recovery from polymyositis or dermatomyositis is estimated to be around 20%, but one thing that experts all seem to agree on is that the earlier the conditions are diagnosed and treated, the better the likely outcome. Although the role of pregnancy in these diseases is not known, either can occur during pregnancy or during the six-week period following birth, and how severe the condition is appears to reflect on the eventual outcome. Essentially, the more active the disease, the greater the chance that the pregnancy will end in miscarriage or stillbirth.

Pseudogout

Understanding the Condition

Pseudogout is a similar form of arthritis to gout, but instead of uric acid crystals forming in the joints, the crystals in pseudogout are made up either of a salt called calcium pyrophosphate dihydrate, or CPPD for short, or apatite, which is a mixture of various calcium phosphate crystals. As crystals develop in the knees, wrists, ankles and other joints, pain and swelling similar to that in gout are experienced. As with gout, pseudogout is characterised by bouts of symptoms which might last for days or weeks, interspersed with periods during which the joints return to normal, often quite spontaneously and without treatment.

The crystals which are formed in pseudogout either develop in the cartilage within the joint or in the tendons which connect muscles to bones. Where the cartilage is affected, the knees are most at risk, but wrists, shoulders and other joints may also be impacted by the disease. In the case of apatite crystal deposits in the tendons, it is the shoulders which are most prone, but again, the hips, hands and other joints can also be affected.

The crystal deposits which characterise pseudogout, although they have the potential to cause severe pain and inflammation, do not always, however, result in symptoms. As is illustrated in Figure 3.10, typically, the crystals are buried quite deeply into the cartilage or tendon and so do not interfere with the workings of the joint. When they move into the joint cavity or into the soft tissues surrounding a tendon, however, their rough, abrasive surfaces can damage cells and cause sudden and extremely painful attacks of inflammation. In addition, because the crystals carry a strong electrical charge, they also have the ability to trigger off the body's defence mechanisms and a pro-inflammatory response. Although in many cases there does not appear to be any apparent reason for crystals to be shed into the joint cavity or soft tissues, sometimes it can be the result of an injury, illness, operation or a heart attack.

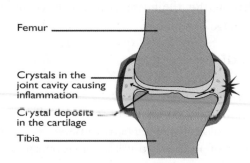

Femur

Crystals in the joint cavity causing inflammation

Crystal deposits in the cartilage

Tibia

Figure 3.10 Shedding of crystals from cartilage into the joint capsule

In those who suffer additionally from osteoarthritis, the presence of these abrasive crystals not only tends to aggravate the sensations of pain and stiffness, but it also contributes to the wearing of cartilage and the thickening of bone which are both characteristic of the disease.

In cases where calcium pyrophosphate crystals affect the cartilage within the joints, an attack of pseudogout typically begins very suddenly and often reaches a peak within as little as 6–12 hours. Only one joint is usually affected, most often the knee, and during the attack this will become hot, swollen and very tender to the touch. As fluid collects in the joint, pressure builds up, causing tension and stiffness in the joint and making it extremely painful to move. As the swelling stretches the skin, the joint also often looks red and shiny. In many cases, these symptoms are also accompanied by fever and a general feeling of being unwell, but usually the swelling starts to die down within about a week, although two to three weeks is normal for the joint to return entirely to normal.

Pseudogout which is caused by apatite crystals and affects the tendons within the joint tends to manifest itself in similar ways to that caused by calcium pyrophosphate crystals, with the main differences being that the swelling tends to occur around the joints rather than inside them and that parts of the body other than the knee are affected. In this case, the shoulder is particularly prone, causing pain over the upper arm and shoulder which is aggravated by raising the arm outwards. Symptoms of swelling, redness and tenderness over the shoulder, and sometimes into the upper arm, again develop quickly, peaking within 12–36 hours. With this type of pseudogout, it is not unknown for the bursa (the fluid-filled sac which sits between the bone and muscle) to burst, causing bruising in the arm which may extend as far down as the elbow. Again, the symptoms tend to settle down gradually on their own, but generally it takes two to four weeks before the area returns to normal.

As with all of the body's systems, balance is crucial for normal functioning and, in the case of pseudogout caused by calcium pyrophosphate crystals, it is an imbalance between the substances which promote and inhibit crystal formation which is responsible for the disease. As this balance alters as we grow older, so the condition appears most frequently in those over the age of 60, with cases in those who are younger than this being rare. With the form of the disease caused by apatite crystals, however, it tends to be younger adults who are most commonly affected. In neither case are men or women more prone.

In most cases, the underlying reasons why crystals develop is not known, but some believe that a genetic abnormality may be responsible for the over production of calcium pyrophosphate and there is certainly some evidence to suggest that pseudogout runs in families. A severely underactive thyroid (hypothyroidism), excess iron storage (haemochromatosis) or magnesium deficiency, however, may also account for the disruption to the regulation of calcium levels and excess calcium in the blood. In some cases involving the formation of apatite crystals in the tendons, diabetes or kidney malfunction may also be the cause.

Diagnosis

Because the symptoms of pseudogout are very similar to those of gout and the condition may even be confused with an infection in the joint, a conclusive diagnosis is normally made by taking a sample of synovial fluid from the joint and subjecting it to microscopic analysis which is aimed at identifying the presence of crystals. As the characteristics of calcium and uric acid crystals are quite different, they are easily distinguishable and so this type of test can readily identify pseudogout as distinct from gout. In some cases, however, both conditions can co-exist and the laboratory test will reveal both types.

In order to rule out the possibility of a joint infection, doctors will often carry out blood tests as part of their investigations, and these are also useful to highlight any elevation in calcium levels, as well as to ensure that the kidneys are functioning normally. In the case of younger patients (i.e. those under the age of 55) or those in whom multiple joints are affected, further blood tests may also be taken to rule in or out any underlying problems which may have contributed to the formation of the crystal deposits.

Unlike with gout, X-rays can be very useful tools where pseudogout is suspected, because these can show up calcification in cartilage and tendons. In some cases, X-rays are repeated several weeks apart to determine whether there has been any decrease in calcification.

Treatment

Despite being a very painful condition during the course of an attack, once a bout of pseudogout is over, there is usually no need for longer term treatment. Seeking treatment for repeated attacks, however, is important, because without this permanent joint damage is a possibility. Even in acute cases though, there is much that can be done to alleviate pain and inflammation and to shorten the length of the attack.

Over-the-counter pain medications such as paracetamol are sometimes helpful in relieving pain, but often stronger prescription drugs which contain codeine are more effective. Non-steroidal anti-inflammatory drugs (NSAIDs), meanwhile, can help with both pain and inflammation and even simple ice packs applied to the affected joint(s) can provide significant relief.

One of the quickest ways to alleviate the pain of pseudogout is through joint aspiration. The drawing off of the fluid immediately reduces the pressure in the joint and may be followed by a long-acting steroid injection which helps to reduce inflammation, as well as preventing the build-up of more fluid. Occasionally, a technique known as lavage may also be carried out in hospital, and this essentially involves washing out the affected joint to remove loose debris.

In cases where attacks of pseudogout are repeated and particularly troublesome, doctors may prescribe low doses of colchicine to reduce the severity and frequency of attacks. Where very large crystals have formed in tendons and the swelling causes tendons to become trapped when the joint is moved, surgery may be considered to remove the deposits.

As we have seen, in the case of gout, diet is absolutely crucial in terms of preventing the build-up of uric acid and the formation of uric acid crystals. In pseudogout, however, the production of calcium pyrophosphate or apatite crystals appears to be largely unaffected by what the individual eats or drinks. Only in those cases where there is an underlying kidney problem or magnesium deficiency would a special diet be recommended therefore. What is important with this condition, however, is that regular exercise is undertaken as soon as the symptoms have been brought under control, as this not only helps to strengthen and prevent wastage of the muscles surrounding the affected joint, but also to assist the inflamed tissues in returning to normal. As part of a multidisciplinary treatment programme, a physiotherapist will be able to advise on the type of exercises which will contribute to recovery without causing further damage.

Psoriatic Arthritis

Understanding the Condition

Psoriatic arthritis is another inflammatory form of the disease, but this time it is associated with the skin condition known as psoriasis. Although not always true, in most cases the arthritis develops after the psoriasis.

Affecting an estimated 2–3% of the population of the UK, psoriasis is an autoimmune disease in which the immune system sends out faulty messages which cause the skin cells to be replaced too quickly. While cells normally replace themselves every three to four weeks, in a patient with psoriasis they will be replaced every two to six days which, in the case of common plaque psoriasis or psoriasis vulgaris (the most common of five different types of the disease), results in the formation of raised red patches covered by silvery-white accumulations of skin on the skin's surface as seen in Figure 3.11.

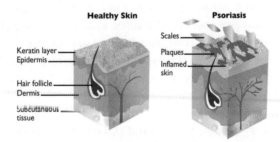

Figure 3.11 Comparison of healthy skin with skin affected by psoriasis

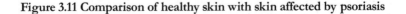

The redness is caused by the increase in blood vessels to support the increased production of cells, and the silvery-white scales are basically skin cells which are waiting to be shed. In common plaque psoriasis, it is most often the elbows, knees, lower back and scalp which are affected, but in fact the disease can affect any area of the body, even the genitals.

Psoriasis can affect people of any age, from children through to the elderly, and approximately one-third of patients are believed to be diagnosed before the age of 20. The disease also has no particular gender preference and affects roughly the same amount of men as women. Although commonly thought to be a contagious disease, this is not the case, and in fact not only can the condition not be passed from one person to another, it cannot be transferred from one area of a sufferer's body to another.

The Psoriasis Association estimates that 5–7% of people with psoriasis also have psoriatic arthritis, but this figure can increase to 40% in the group of people who have severe psoriasis. Like psoriasis itself, psoriatic arthritis affects men and women equally and can appear at any age, although the majority of cases are diagnosed in those between the ages of 30 and 50. In 70% of cases, the psoriasis comes first, in 15% the psoriatic arthritis comes first and in the remaining 15% the two conditions appear at the same time, but it is also worth noting that sufferers of psoriasis can also develop other forms of arthritis such as osteoarthritis and rheumatoid arthritis, although these are not linked to the skin disease.

Psoriatic arthritis most commonly affects the joints of the hands and the feet (particularly the small joints closest to the ends of the fingers and toes), but it can also produce pain, inflammation and swelling in the neck, wrists, shoulders and ankles, as well as the larger joints of the body such as the knees, elbows, hips and spine. In some cases the condition might be mild with only a few joints being affected, whereas in others it could be much more severe and involve many joints. The most severe and destructive form of psoriatic arthritis, arthritis mutilans, often leads to a significant and marked deformity of the joints. Typically though, the symptoms of the arthritis will come and go along with the symptoms of the psoriasis itself, and might include:

- Pain, stiffness, swelling, throbbing and tenderness in the affected joints
- Decreased range of movement in the affected joints
- Pain, swelling and tenderness in the area of the tendons
- Swelling of entire fingers and toes (known as dactylitis)
- General fatigue
- Changes in the nails to give a pitted appearance or which cause the nail to become separated from the nail bed

Where psoriatic arthritis affects the spine, stiffness and pain which are most commonly experienced in the lower back towards the base of the spine or the neck are often the first signs of the condition.

Although psoriatic arthritis does not normally affect organs such as the lungs, kidneys or liver, it is thought that those who suffer from the condition may have a greater tendency to develop heart disease. Stopping smoking, keeping alcohol consumption to a minimum and controlling weight, as well as dealing with high blood pressure, therefore, are all important for those with the condition. In addition, sufferers can find themselves prone to frequent bouts of conjunctivitis (inflammation of the inside of the eyelid and of the membrane covering the front of the eye) and/or iritis (inflammation of the iris), for which treatment should be sought.

Diagnosis

Diagnosing psoriatic arthritis is not always easy, firstly because there is no specific test for the condition and secondly because it is sometimes not easily distinguishable from rheumatoid arthritis. Generally, diagnosis is made based on the patient's description of his or her symptoms and on physical examination, and of course if the patient's medical history indicates that psoriasis runs in the family, this too will provide important clues. Doctors pay particularly close attention to how the disease presents itself and which joints are affected, as psoriatic arthritis tends to present in one of five distinguishable patterns. Although blood tests may be carried out, these are done purely to rule out other forms of the disease, rather than to conclusively identify the psoriatic form, but joint X-rays can be helpful because the effects of psoriatic arthritis tend to show up differently than with other types of the disease.

Because the onset and progression of psoriatic arthritis is sometimes quite subtle, it does have the potential to develop into quite a serious condition if it is not detected and treated early. Although there is currently no known prevention or cure for the disease, a multidisciplinary approach which also aims to treat the associated skin condition can do much to alleviate pain and discomfort.

Treatment

Pain-relieving medications, as well as non-steroidal anti-inflammatory drugs (NSAIDs) typically represent a first line of attack against psoriatic arthritis, but often more severe cases also require more powerful medication in the form of disease-modifying anti-rheumatic drugs (DMARDs) such as methotrexate (sold under brand names such as Rheumatrex and Trexall) and sulfasalazine (branded as Salazopyrine in Europe and Azulfidine in the US). TNF (tumour necrosis factor) inhibitors have also been found to be helpful in some cases of psoriasis and psoriatic arthritis, as well as in some involving rheumatoid arthritis and ankylosing spondylitis. These drugs effectively inhibit the body's inflammatory response but, like many medications, they do have the potential to present some significant side effects.

Along with oral medications, steroid injections can also provide effective relief for joints which are particularly painful, but a range of non-invasive therapies such as heat and cold therapies typically prove to be extremely helpful too. Physical therapies, exercise and diet, meanwhile, form important parts of a multidisciplinary treatment programme as these help to improve and maintain strength and mobility, as well as reducing the strain which is exerted on the joints.

The treatments for psoriasis which are ideally carried out in conjunction with those for psoriatic arthritis as part of a holistic treatment regime might include topical treatments (creams and ointments which are applied directly to the skin), phototherapy (exposure of the skin to certain types of ultraviolet light) or medication which is aimed at slowing down the rate at which skin cells are replaced or targeting specific parts of the immune system. Medication may be taken orally or administered by injection as appropriate.

Although psoriatic arthritis can sometimes be severe in terms of the pain and immobility that it produces, as well as in terms of the deformities that it can cause, the effects of the disease are often mild and joint replacement surgery is rarely required. What does make this form of the disease particularly distressing for sufferers, however, is the fact that patients have to endure not only the painful joint disease, but the severe discomfort and physical disfigurement of the skin condition too. Where emotional and psychological problems develop as a result of either or both of the diseases, these too can be tackled as part of a holistic treatment programme.

Reactive Arthritis

Understanding the Condition
Not to be confused with septic arthritis, reactive arthritis (also known as Reiter's syndrome) is a condition in which inflammation of the joints occurs as a reaction to an earlier infection elsewhere in the body. Usually it affects the knees, ankles and toes, but the elbows, wrists and fingers, as well as the joints at the base of the spine, can also become inflamed.

Most common in people between the ages of 20 and 40, reactive arthritis is estimated to affect only 30–40 out of every 100,000 people in England each year. The infections which cause the condition are usually sexually transmitted infections such as chlamydia, or the types of infections of the gut which commonly cause food poisoning. In fact, Arthritis Research UK estimates that 1–2% of people who experience food poisoning go on to suffer joint inflammation afterwards. While 90% of cases involving reactive arthritis as the result of a sexually transmitted infection are believed to involve men, both men and women are equally prone to those caused by infections of the bowel and gut.

The severity of the symptoms of reactive arthritis varies hugely from one person to another and although pain and swelling of the joints are often some of the first signs of the condition, as you can see from Figure 3.12, this form of arthritis can also cause:

■ Conjunctivitis (inflammation of the eyes)
■ Mouth ulcers

- Diarrhoea, which may be present before the joint symptoms
- Skin lesions on the palms of the hands and soles of the feet
- Urethritis (inflammation of the tube which runs from the bladder to where urine exits the body)

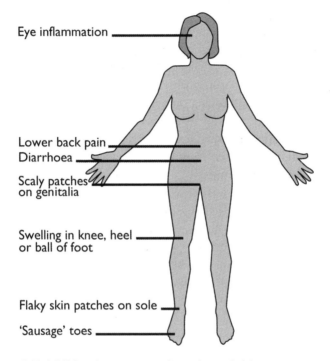

Figure 3.12 Additional symptoms of reactive arthritis

The skin lesions which are sometimes characteristic of reactive arthritis are known as keratoderma blennorrhagica and they typically resemble the scaly skin rashes which are associated with psoriasis. Although most commonly found on the palms and soles, they can spread to the scrotum, scalp and trunk. In men, reactive arthritis can also produce a painful rash which appears at the end of the penis. The swelling of the fingers or toes which is known in medical terms as dactylitis but commonly called 'sausage toes' or 'sausage fingers', meanwhile, occurs when not only the joint itself becomes inflamed, but also the tendons which sit around the joint.

Unlike some of the more chronic types of arthritis, reactive arthritis usually tends to disappear within 12 months, with some cases taking as little as three months to resolve themselves and the majority taking six. Only rarely does the condition become more persistent and require long-term treatment.

Diagnosis

Although there is no specific test which can be used to diagnose reactive arthritis, a thorough patient history can often help to identify a link to an earlier infection. Even if this is not the case, the combination of symptoms which tend to be present with this form of arthritis can provide tremendous clues as to the source of the problem. If the disease is suspected, blood tests can often be helpful in ruling out other types of arthritis, such as rheumatoid arthritis, and swabs taken from the penis or vagina can be used to confirm that there are indeed signs of inflammation or infection.

Treatment

Although reactive arthritis is a condition which occurs as the result of an earlier infection elsewhere in the body other than the joints, in some cases that infection may still be present. If this is the case, one of the first courses of action would be to treat it with antibiotics. Further to this, however, non-steroidal anti-inflammatory drugs (NSAIDs) and painkillers may be prescribed to reduce joint swelling and help to alleviate pain symptoms. If the inflammation is severe, steroid injections may also be an option and if the case of reactive arthritis is more persistent and long-lasting, disease-modifying anti-rheumatic drugs (DMARDs) may be recommended.

Both if the body is still trying to fight the original infection which caused the reactive arthritis or if the joint inflammation itself is active, it is quite likely that the sufferer will feel tired and generally unwell. While it is important to exercise the joints in order to maintain mobility and muscle strength, rest also has an important part to play in recovering from this form of the disease, particularly in the early days. Of course, for those who are prone to bouts of food poisoning or whose lifestyles put them at greater risk of sexually transmitted infections, special care needs to be taken to avoid a recurrence of the condition.

Septic Arthritis

Understanding the Condition

As I have just said, reactive arthritis is a form of the disease in which the joints are affected by earlier infection elsewhere in the body. Septic arthritis, on the other hand, is an active infection within the joint itself.

Also known as infectious arthritis, septic arthritis can be caused by bacteria, viruses or fungi, and microorganisms can either spread to the joint through the bloodstream when there is infection present elsewhere in the body, or they can enter the joint through a wound or during surgery. It is not only 'natural' joints which can be affected by this type of arthritis, but prosthetic joints too. In the latter case, an abscess may develop around the joint or the implant may become loose. Although a variety of microorganisms can be responsible for causing septic arthritis, the most common culprit is the bacterium *Staphylococcus aureus*, and this and the *Streptococcus* bacterium generally cause some of the most sudden and severe cases of the condition.

Because of the way that septic arthritis develops, certain groups of people are more at risk than others, including those who:

- Have sustained an injury
- Have undergone surgery
- Have an infection of the bone (osteomyelitis) close to a joint
- Are involved in intravenous drug abuse
- Suffer from immune deficiency disorders
- Are taking medications which suppress the immune system
- Have suffered joint disease in the past
- Have underlying medical conditions such as diabetes, sickle cell disease or rheumatic diseases such as rheumatoid arthritis
- Are alcoholic
- Have an artificial joint, such as a hip or knee

Although septic arthritis can affect a number of joints in the body, it is more common for only one to become infected and in around 50% of cases it is the knee. The hip joints, meanwhile, account for around 20% of cases, the shoulders 8% and the ankles and wrists each 7%. Symptoms of the condition normally develop quite quickly, often within just a few days, although where an artificial joint is affected, the signs may appear more gradually.

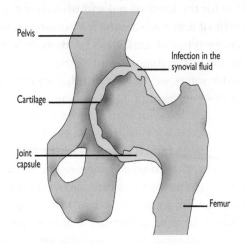

Pelvis

Infection in the synovial fluid

Cartilage

Joint capsule

Femur

Figure 3.13 Hip joint affected by septic arthritis

As you can see from Figure 3.13 which depicts a hip joint affected by septic arthritis, the synovial fluid within the joint becomes infected, which in turn typically causes symptoms which may include:

- Severe joint pain
- Swelling caused by an abnormal build-up of joint fluid
- Stiffness of the joint
- Redness and warmth of the joint
- Joint tenderness
- The inability to move the limb with the infected joint (known as pseudoparalysis)
- Fever
- Chills
- Feeling of being generally unwell

Diagnosis
Although septic arthritis is not a common condition, it can however be quite serious and so needs to be treated without delay. Blood tests and cultures are normally used to diagnose the presence

of inflammation in the body and may help to determine the presence and type of microorganism. A sample of synovial fluid may also be taken from the joint and this will be checked for colour and clarity, as well as for the levels of red and white blood cells and for bacteria. The type of bacteria is important because some strains are resistant to certain types of antibiotics. Although X-rays are not particularly useful in the diagnosis of septic arthritis, especially during the earlier stages of the condition, they can help to rule out other causes of joint pain.

Treatment

Because septic arthritis is caused by infection, the first line of attack is antibiotics and these are often administered intravenously and at high doses in the first instance and then followed up with doses to be taken orally. Even if the type of bacteria has not yet been identified through laboratory tests, antibiotics which are used to treat the forms which most commonly cause the condition will be tried first and then the medication adjusted if the test results reveal a different strain. Usually the antibiotics will act quickly in the system and symptoms will begin to die down within just a few days.

Another thing which is particularly important in the treatment of septic arthritis is the drainage of infected fluid from the joint to avoid any lasting damage. With knees, elbows, shoulders, ankles and wrists, this can normally be done fairly easily using a needle, but in the case of deeper joints such as the hips, it may require a small operation. In either case, fluid drainage may have to be performed several times until the build-up of infected fluid stops. In cases where an artificial joint becomes infected, the joint may have to be removed in order for it to be treated properly, but in most cases a replacement can be fitted without any problem.

While the infection is being treated, cool compresses may help to relieve pain, and rest and immobilisation of the affected joint is typically necessary. In some cases, the joint may need to be splinted to avoid the pain of movement. As soon as possible after the symptoms have begun to settle, however, physiotherapy is important to mobilise the joint, promote healing and prevent any long-term stiffness.

The prognosis for sufferers of septic arthritis is generally good if the infection is treated swiftly, and often there are no long-term after-effects. If treatment is delayed, however, parts of the joint can quickly be destroyed, with long-term pain, restricted joint mobility and even some degree of disability being the result. Should the infection be severe and go undiagnosed, there is also the risk of septicaemia (blood poisoning) which can be fatal, although modern antibiotics make this a much rarer occurrence than in years gone by.

Scleroderma

Understanding the Condition

As I said at the start of this book, the term 'arthritis' covers more than 100 different diseases, all of which affect the joints in one way or another. In some cases the joint symptoms are predominant, while in others they appear as secondary to other effects or develop as only one of a wide range of symptoms. In scleroderma, the most obvious effects of the condition appear on the skin, and in fact the name of the disease actually means 'hard skin'.

Scleroderma manifests itself in two quite distinct forms:

■ Localised scleroderma, in which only parts of the skin and underlying tissues, and sometimes the underlying muscles are affected, and

■ Systemic scleroderma, in which the joints, muscles, blood vessels and digestive system are affected, and occasionally the heart, lungs and kidneys

Localised Scleroderma

Because the effects of localised scleroderma are limited and the condition rarely progresses to the systemic form, this is considered to be the less serious of the two forms of the disease. It can be sub-divided into two different types, known as morphoea scleroderma and linear scleroderma. In the former, there may be one or more localised patches of hard, reddened skin which are white at the centre and purplish in colour around the outside, or the patches may extend over much larger areas and indeed over most or all of the body. These lesions can appear anywhere on the body and they can remain active for anywhere from a few weeks to several years, after which time the skin starts to soften, although often leaving a darkened patch. In the case of linear scleroderma, as the name suggests there is a single line or band of thickened and discoloured skin which typically runs down the arm or leg, although it can also appear on the forehead.

Systemic Scleroderma

Systemic scleroderma, which is the type that doctors are usually describing when they use the general term, typically affects a number of the body's systems. This form can also be sub-divided into two different types:

- Limited systemic scleroderma, in which the thickening and discolouration of the skin is limited to the fingers, forearm, face, neck and legs. In this case, the likelihood of any major effects on the internal organs is only slim, but the symptoms of calcinosis, Raynaud's phenomenon, oesophageal dysmotility, sclerodactyly and telangiectasia (known by the acronym CREST) may all be experienced
- Diffuse systemic scleroderma, in which skin thickening and discolouration may appear anywhere on the body and in which significant organ involvement normally follows shortly after the onset of Raynaud's phenomenon. In this form of the condition, it is during the first three to five years that most damage to the body is likely to occur, after which time the disease tends to settle down, with any effects on the skin or the organs slowing down or stopping entirely. Eventually, the skin then begins to soften and further serious damage to the organs becomes less likely

As mentioned above, systemic scleroderma can present with a number of symptoms. As each case is unique, however, both the form and the severity of the condition will determine precisely which are experienced and to what extent. Here though, are the main ones associated with the disease.

- Changes to the skin – skin changes tend to manifest themselves early on in the course of the disease, with mild inflammation and swelling initially causing the skin to tighten and flexibility to become compromised. With the progression of the disease, not only does the skin become thicker, but the oil and sweat glands stop functioning so that the skin dries out and becomes itchy. This stage of the condition normally lasts for one to three years before the skin starts to soften and grow thinner.

■ Raynaud's phenomenon – Raynaud's phenomenon is a condition in which cold temperatures or emotional distress causes the blood vessels in the hands and/or feet to become constricted, and it is one which is believed to affect more than 90% of scleroderma sufferers. Often it is the first sign of the disease and manifests itself quite obviously as the hands or feet start to feel cold before going very pale and then turning blue. Usually within 10–15 minutes, the blood vessels open up again, causing the skin to turn red and mottled-looking, but with repeated attacks, the condition can cause skin ulcers to develop on the fingertips.

■ Calcinosis – calcinosis occurs when calcium deposits form either underneath the skin or within the muscles. These deposits can cause repeated bouts of inflammation on the skin which covers them or they can lead to skin ulcers.

■ Oesophageal dysmotility – the purpose of the oesophagus is essentially to ensure that food is efficiently delivered from the mouth to the stomach, but in the case of an oesophageal dysmotility disorder, this process is disrupted when the smooth muscles lose their ability to move normally. This can either mean that the food is prevented from reaching the stomach or that it is regurgitated, and the symptoms which are typical include chronic heartburn and chest pain, pain or difficulty in swallowing or the feeling of having a permanent lump in the throat.

■ Sclerodactyly – sclerodactyly is the term which is used to describe the thickening of the skin on the digits of the hands or feet.

■ Telangiectasia – telangiectasia is a condition in which small dilated blood vessels appear near the surface of the skin. Although the condition is not a dangerous one, the fact that the vessels can be seen through the skin can give an unsightly appearance.

■ Arthralgia and myalgia – arthralgia is basically pain in the joints which can occur as the result of a number of different causes, and myalgia refers to pain in the muscles. Both pain and stiffness commonly occur in patients of systemic scleroderma in the early stages of the disease, and often this develops into muscle weakness and wastage later on.

■ Problems of the mouth or teeth – problems with the mouth or teeth can develop in one of two ways. First of all, the patient may suffer Sjögren's syndrome secondary to systemic scleroderma and suffer dryness of the mouth due to inflammation of the salivary glands. The lack of saliva production can then in turn lead to tooth decay, gum disease and mouth sores, and ultimately affect the patient's ability to chew or to take in sufficient quantities of nutrients. In addition, if the skin around the mouth becomes tight, it may not be possible to open the mouth very wide, which can again have an effect on the ability to maintain good oral hygiene and lead to dental problems.

■ Gastrointestinal problems – as well as affecting the oesophagus, systemic scleroderma can also cause problems along the whole of the gastrointestinal tract, leading to an abnormal backward flow of body fluids known as reflux, nausea, vomiting, bloating, abdominal cramps, diarrhoea, weight loss and, ultimately, malnutrition.

■ Kidney disease – where serious kidney disease occurs as the result of systemic scleroderma, the symptoms most often show up within the first four to five years of the disease. High blood pressure, along with rapidly progressive kidney failure are the most characteristic signs of kidney disease, which tends to occur most often in those with the diffuse form of the condition.

■ Heart disease – heart disease does not usually manifest itself except in more advanced cases of systemic scleroderma, and then the symptoms typically include shortness of breath (usually after some form of exertion), heart palpitations and, occasionally, chest pain.

■ Lung disease – of all the symptoms of systemic scleroderma, lung disease has the greatest potential to lead to fatality, making the testing of lung function vital for early detection. Symptoms normally begin with breathing difficulties, either spontaneously or following some kind of exertion, but can progress to hardening of the lung tissue (pulmonary fibrosis) and high blood pressure in the artery which carries blood from the heart to the lungs (pulmonary hypertension).

In addition to these quite specific symptoms, sufferers of systemic scleroderma might also experience other signs, such as:

■ Fatigue
■ Appetite and weight loss
■ Swelling of the hands and feet, especially in the mornings
■ Shiny skin which looks stretched and without its normal creases
■ Thinning of the skin on the fingertips
■ Sexual dysfunction or impotence
■ Depression
■ Thyroid disorders
■ Sjögren's syndrome
■ Carpal tunnel syndrome

As can be seen from Figure 3.14, contracture (or the tightening into a bent position) of some joints can occur. Often it is the fingers which are affected and this stage of the disease is typically followed by the thinning of the skin on the fingertips.

Normal
hand

Hand affected
by scleroderma

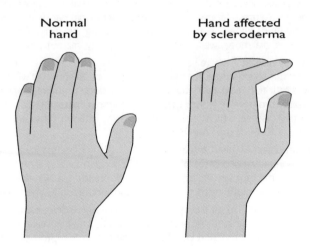

Figure 3.14 Hand affected by scleroderma

Scleroderma is a long-term or chronic disease which normally starts between the ages of 25 and 55 but can also affect children and older people. According to Arthritis Research UK, women are three to four times more likely to suffer from the condition than men, but it is nevertheless a rare disease.

Although it is not known precisely why, those affected by scleroderma produce too much collagen in their bodies. Collagen is the main component of the connective tissues which hold our bodies together and so is essential, but when too much of it is produced, the tissues become stiff and hard, the skin becomes tight and the internal organs are unable to function properly. While some believe that the condition is an autoimmune disorder, others suspect that the predominance of the disease in women of childbearing age is accounted for by a connection with the hormone oestrogen. Although there appears to be no direct genetic link, genes may play a role in setting up a predisposition to the illness, which could then be triggered by certain environmental factors such as different chemicals or even certain viruses.

Diagnosis

Diagnosis of scleroderma begins, as with other forms of arthritis, with the taking of the patient's full medical history and a physical examination. Because this particular disease can take some considerable time for some of the symptoms to develop, however, it can be months before other conditions can be ruled out and a conclusive diagnosis arrived at. The thickening of the skin, however, is of course a tell-tale sign of the condition and so is often a key factor in identifying the disease, although doctors will often carry out other tests such as blood tests, X-rays, skin biopsies, heart scans and breathing tests to help them determine whether other parts of the body have been affected.

Treatment

Although there is no cure for scleroderma, doctors can prescribe a number of different drugs to help control the various symptoms. Amongst these, non-steroidal anti-inflammatory drugs (NSAIDs) can be useful in relieving pain and inflammation in the joints, while medications such as angiotensin-converting enzyme (ACE) inhibitors and calcium channel blockers can help to lower blood pressure and improve blood circulation. Nifedipine can also be used to help widen the blood vessels and so reduce the effects of Raynaud's phenomenon. Where problems of the digestive system arise or if severe heartburn is an issue, antacids can help to alleviate these symptoms, and creams and infusions may be recommended to treat skin ulcers. Low-dosage steroids and immunosuppressant drugs, meanwhile, can prove especially helpful in cases where the lungs are affected or where the effects on the skin are more considerable. Steroids may also be used to treat muscle pain.

In addition to using the treatments recommended by doctors, sufferers of scleroderma can do much to limit the pain and discomfort which is caused by the various symptoms of the disease, including:

- Taking regular exercise to improve blood flow, maintain elasticity in the skin and stop the joints from tightening up
- Stopping smoking. Smoking causes the blood vessels to narrow and so aggravates the symptoms of Raynaud's phenomenon

- Avoiding the cold and dressing warmly in layers
- Applying moisturising creams and lotions frequently, especially after bathing
- Using sunscreen
- Avoiding harsh detergents or chemicals or using rubber gloves to protect the skin if this is not possible
- Using warm rather than hot water for baths or showers
- Using dressings to protect sore or broken skin
- Taking frequent sips of water or chewing sugarless gum to keep the mouth moist
- Ensuring good oral hygiene
- Eating small and frequent meals and avoiding late-night meals to help counter gastrointestinal problems

As stress can not only affect the blood flow to certain parts of the body, but also create muscle tension which leads to increased levels of pain, a multidisciplinary treatment programme should also seek to teach relaxation techniques and to address any underlying issues which might be contributing to anxiety or depression.

Spondyloarthritis

As I mentioned at the beginning of the section on Juvenile Spondyloarthritis, spondyloarthritis which begins before the age of 16 is known as juvenile spondyloarthritis, but the condition can also affect those in their adult years. Most often it is people between the ages of 20 and 30 who are diagnosed with the condition.

Spondyloarthritis which occurs in adults is essentially the same as that which affects children. Not only does the term encompass the same range of arthritic conditions as with the childhood form of the disease, but the same range of possible symptoms, methods of diagnosis, treatments and considerations all apply too.

Systemic Lupus Erythematosus

Understanding the Condition
Systemic lupus erythematosus, which is commonly abbreviated to SLE or just lupus, is a chronic, non-contagious, incurable and sometimes disabling autoimmune disease which can be extremely

dangerous, particularly in cases where complications arise. The condition affects the skin, joints and sometimes the internal organs such as the heart and lungs and, being one of two forms of lupus, it should not be confused with discoid lupus which only affects the skin.

Unlike some forms of arthritis which tend to affect older people, SLE is far more common in younger females. Around 3 out of every 10,000 people in the UK are believed to suffer from the condition, with nine times more women than men falling prey to the disease, the majority of whom are of child bearing age. According to Arthritis Research UK, only 1 in every 15 cases begins after the age of 50 and these tend to be much less severe. While children can also suffer from SLE, the condition is quite rare in youngsters and the Arthritis Foundation in the USA reports that around 25,000 children and adolescents in the country have lupus or a related disorder.

The reason why antibodies attack otherwise healthy body tissues in lupus is unknown, but it is believed that environmental or hormonal factors may play a part in the onset of the condition. Genes which are passed down through families may also be responsible for the development of SLE, although the condition is not directly inherited from one's parents.

Although it does have certain characteristic features, SLE can sometimes be quite difficult for doctors to diagnose in its early stages as many of the symptoms are not dissimilar to those of flu, including:

- Fever
- Low energy levels
- Appetite loss, and
- Widespread aches and pains

As time goes on and the disease progresses, however, further symptoms such as those highlighted in Figure 3.15 become apparent, although precisely which ones are experienced and at what level of severity can vary enormously from person to person.

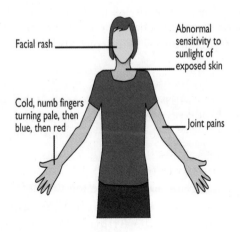

Facial rash

Abnormal
sensitivity to
sunlight of
exposed skin

Cold, numb fingers
turning pale, then
blue, then red

Joint pains

Figure 3.15 Key symptoms of SLE

Some of the most common areas of the body to be affected include:

- The skin – one of the most common and characteristic symptoms of SLE is a butterfly-shaped rash which appears across the cheeks and the bridge of the nose, and in fact it is partly this rash to which the condition owes its name. 'Lupus' is actually the Latin word for 'wolf' and it was because the rash was reminiscent of the white markings on a wolf's face that the condition earned its name. It is not only the face which can be affected however, and the rash may also appear on the chest, hands, wrists or other parts of the body, particularly after exposure to the sun. In some cases, patients may also experience the symptoms of Raynaud's phenomenon in which the hands and feet are affected by cold and in which the colour of the skin changes from white to blue to red.

- The mouth – people who suffer from SLE are often plagued with mouth ulcers which typically appear in groups and come and go. Around 12% of sufferers also exhibit symptoms of Sjögren's syndrome, another autoimmune disorder which in this case causes the immune system to attack the tear and salivary glands, causing dryness of the mouth and eyes.

- The hair – hair loss is quite common in sufferers of SLE. Although in many cases it is not significant and only amounts to a thinning of the hair, some patients do experience significant hair loss. The hair does normally grow back during periods when the disease is less active however.

■ The joints – pain and swelling in the joints are sometimes the primary symptoms of SLE and usually it is the small joints in the hands and feet which are primarily affected. In most cases, however, there is no permanent damage to or deformity of the joints and only around 5% of sufferers can expect to experience more severe or lasting joint problems.

■ The blood and lymphatic systems – SLE can cause high blood pressure to develop, particularly when the disease affects the kidneys, as well as mild anaemia as the result of effects on the bone marrow. In rare cases it can also affect the ability of the blood to clot or create a tendency for blood clots to form. Sometimes the condition can cause painful swelling of the lymph glands and sometimes the steroids which are used to treat SLE are responsible for the elevation in blood pressure.

■ The kidneys – around one-third of people with SLE develop inflammation of the kidneys which can lead to blood and proteins being leaked into the urine. This is not normally a serious complication of the condition and does not usually cause any particular problems. Kidney failure is very rare.

■ The heart and lungs – although the actual tissues of the heart and lungs themselves are rarely affected in SLE, sometimes there is inflammation in the tissues which line these organs. In the case of the heart, this can cause pericarditis and sharp pains in the centre of the chest and, where the lungs are affected, breathlessness develops as the result of pleurisy. On rare occasions, severe breathlessness can occur if large amounts of fluid develop in lining tissues.

■ The brain and nervous system – around one in three SLE sufferers develop migraines as a result of the condition and normal headaches are quite common. Although quite rare, some also experience fits which are similar to those in epilepsy. What are fairly typical with SLE, however, are feelings of depression and anxiety, but it is not certain whether these are actually features of the disease itself or whether they occur as a reaction to the fear and hopelessness of suffering from a chronic illness.

Although mild cases of SLE which affect only the joints or the joints and the skin, and moderate cases which also cause some inflammation in other parts of the body can be extremely troublesome, it is only in the more rare and severe cases where the heart, lungs, kidneys or brain are damaged that the condition can potentially become life-threatening. As SLE usually develops quite slowly, however, early diagnosis, treatment and ongoing monitoring usually mean that the disease is controlled before it reaches this stage.

Diagnosis

If a description of symptoms along with a physical examination tends to suggest SLE then doctors normally carry out a range of blood tests to confirm the diagnosis. Although the latter cannot provide 100% conclusive evidence that the condition is present, they can give very strong suggestions that this is the case, as well as helping to distinguish it from other conditions with similar symptoms and heading off any complications of the disease. An anti-nuclear antibody (ANA) test, for example, shows up as positive in 95% of people who suffer from SLE and an anti-DNA antibody test almost never comes back positive for those who are not sufferers of the condition. An erythrocyte sedimentation rate (ESR) test, which measures how quickly blood cells settle in a test tube, meanwhile, is also likely to indicate active SLE, because the cells settle more quickly when the disease is present, and a complement level test which looks at proteins in the blood is likely to show decreased levels. Other blood tests can help to indicate a greater likelihood of Sjögren's syndrome, miscarriage or of developing blood clots, as well as any effects on the bone marrow, liver and kidneys. In fact, many of these tests, along with urine tests, X-rays, ultrasound scans and magnetic resonance imaging (MRI) scans, are not only used to diagnose SLE and the extent of its effects initially, but also as part of the monitoring of patients' conditions and as a means of predicting a flare-up when the disease becomes active after a period of remission.

Treatment

SLE, as I have mentioned, is not a curable condition, but it can be controlled nevertheless. Because each case is unique and a variety of symptoms may present in a variety of different ways, however, treatment programmes must be tailor-made to suit each individual patient.

Some of the drugs used to control SLE act on just one of the symptoms of the condition, whereas others have more than one benefit. Non-steroidal anti-inflammatory drugs (NSAIDs), for example, typically help with joint pain and swelling, while steroids (administered in either injection or tablet form) can be used to combat hair loss and to treat complications such as pleurisy and pericarditis and steroid creams can be used for rashes. Hydroxy-chloroquine, meanwhile, can not only be effective at treating rashes, but also has positive effects on the fatigue that many SLE sufferers experience. As part of a holistic and multidisciplinary treatment regime, a variety of other medications may also be pre-scribed to suppress the immune system and stop it from attacking the body's tissues so aggressively, as well as to reduce the risks of further complications caused by, for example, steroid medications.

In cases where excess fluid builds up in the lining tissues of the heart or lungs, this may need to be drained using a needle and syringe, but only in this case or in the rare event of kidney failure would invasive treatments normally be required. Where joint pain is a particular problem, many patients find that acupuncture is helpful, although it can take a number of treatments before any longer-term benefit is derived.

In addition to the treatments offered by practitioners, sufferers of SLE can also do much to protect themselves from the symptoms or the complications of the condition. Avoiding exposure to the sun, for instance, can stop symptoms from being aggravated, and because the taking of steroids and immunosuppressants can leave SLE patients more prone to infection, avoiding contact with people who have infections can minimise any risk. Women are also advised to discuss contraception with their physicians as some forms of oral contraceptives may not be advisable, depending upon the severity of the disease. Finding the right balance between rest and exercise is also important for sufferers of SLE, as when the disease is active it can often leave the patient feeling starved of energy and disinclined to do very much. While it is important to rest when needed, a total lack of activity can lead to muscle wastage, further joint problems, a decline in overall fitness and stamina and weight gain.

Although the prognosis for those suffering from SLE is very much better than it was years ago and most people only experience a mild form of the condition, severe cases can shorten normal life expectancy and cause disability. Even in the milder cases, however, the impact of dealing with a life-long illness, as well as the effects of the physical disfigurations caused by facial rashes, can make SLE very difficult to live with. As I have mentioned, depression and anxiety are not uncommon in those with the disease, which is one of the reasons why a multidisciplinary approach to treatment which includes a psychotherapeutic element is typically much more effective and appropriate.

Tennis Elbow

Understanding the Condition

Whether tennis elbow is a condition which properly constitutes a form of arthritis is something upon which those in the medical world are not in agreement. As it is another common condition which directly affects the joints, however, I have chosen to include it here.

Tennis elbow is actually the more common name for a condition which is known as lateral epicondylitis, because it affects the lateral epicondyle or the bony lump on the outside of the elbow. Despite its name though, tennis elbow is not just a condition which is caused by playing the sport. In fact, it can be caused by any activity which leads to the overuse of the muscles in the forearm or by a single, forceful injury. Anything which is done regularly such as wringing out washing, typing or using a screwdriver or garden shears, as well as racquet sports and sports which involve throwing, such as javelin or discus, can cause the condition. In some cases, however, damage can occur as the result of lifting something heavy or doing something like painting and decorating which is not normally done very often. Occasionally, there is no history of overuse of the arm or of any prior injury and the condition just seems to develop spontaneously and without any apparent cause.

Tennis elbow affects both men and women equally and around 5 in every 1,000 people develop the condition each year. Although it can affect anyone of any age, it tends to be more common in those between 35 and 60. Often it is those people whose forearm muscles are unfit and who suddenly take part in activities that they are not normally used to who start to experience symptoms. If you suddenly start playing a lot of racquet sports while on holiday, for instance, you could be at greater risk. As might be expected, the condition tends to occur in the dominant arm, but this is not always the case and around 25% of cases are estimated to occur in the non-dominant one.

What actually happens in tennis elbow is that the tendons which attach the muscles and bones in the elbow joint suffer tiny injuries. As can be seen from Figure 3.16, these injuries result in pain and inflammation in the area around the lateral epicondyle on the outer side of the elbow, although the pain can also travel down the forearm towards the wrist. Generally, the area will feel tender to the touch and there may even be some swelling. Tingling in the arm or the fingers, however, is not normally a sign of tennis elbow, and where these symptoms are experienced it is much more likely to be due to a problem with a nerve in the neck or the wrist.

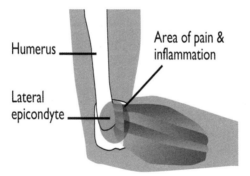

Humerus

Area of pain & inflammation

Lateral epicondyte

Figure 3.16 Area of inflammation caused by tennis elbow

For most people who have tennis elbow, pain is only experienced when the affected forearm or wrist is used, particularly for movements which involve twisting, such as if they were to try to open a jar or turn a doorknob. Often there will also be difficulties in holding items or in straightening the arm fully, and some people also experience stiffness in the affected arm. In some cases, however, the pain is constant and can even interfere with the sufferer's ability to sleep comfortably.

Diagnosis

The diagnosis of tennis elbow is normally very straightforward and is typically based on a description of the symptoms, enquiries into the patient's medical history and a physical examination. In some cases, the doctor may choose to carry out blood tests or X-rays, but this is usually only done to rule out any other possible conditions. Only in rare cases where treatments have failed to deal with the symptoms would an ultrasound scan of the soft tissues in the arm be called for.

Treatment

In many cases, tennis elbow clears up of its own accord without any need for treatment, and avoiding any activities which cause pain and aggravate inflammation can help to speed recovery by allowing the damaged tendon to heal. If pain relief is required in the meantime, ice packs or a hot water bottle applied to the area can be effective and simple painkillers such as ibuprofen and anti-inflammatory gels which are rubbed into the skin can also help. If these are not sufficient, a steroid injection into the tender area may be given, although usually it will still be necessary to rest the affected arm for several weeks afterwards.

Where the pain of tennis elbow is more persistent, physiotherapy such as massage, laser or ultrasound therapy carried out by a trained professional may be beneficial. Some doctors may also prescribe a nitric oxide transdermal patch, as this chemical compound has recently been shown to help with the healing of tendons. Only on rare occasions does tennis elbow necessitate surgery and, if this is the case, a small operation can be carried out to release the affected tendon.

With simple rest and painkillers, tennis elbow will normally settle down within 6 to 12 weeks, although in some cases it might be as little as 3 weeks or as long as up to 2 years. Usually it does not cause any lasting damage to the tendons, but those who have had the condition are more likely to have it again

4

Related and Secondary Medical Conditions

As I mentioned earlier, the conditions that I have talked about in Chapter 3 are all ones which directly and primarily affect the joints of the body and which most doctors would agree can properly be described as forms of arthritis. As you will have seen, however, there are a number of other diseases and disorders which can develop as a result of arthritis, in tandem with it, which can be a precursor to it or are commonly confused with it. In this chapter, therefore, I will take a look at some of those which you will most often hear mentioned in relation to arthritis.

Carpal Tunnel Syndrome

Carpal tunnel syndrome is a condition which generally affects the dominant hand of the sufferer, although it can affect either or both hands. It affects people of all ages, although women tend to be more prone to the condition than men, and it can result from arthritic conditions which impact on the wrist, particularly rheumatoid arthritis.

As can be seen in Figure 4.1, the carpal tunnel is a narrow 'tunnel' in the wrist which is made up of bone on the bottom and sides and ligament across the top. The median nerve, which travels from the forearm into the hand and controls sensations and nerve functions in the hand, passes through the carpal tunnel along with nine tendons which connect muscles to bones and allow the thumb and fingers to bend.

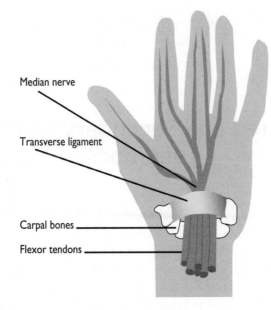

Figure 4.1 Arrangement of the carpal tunnel

What happens in carpal tunnel syndrome is that the median nerve becomes pressed or squeezed where it passes through this narrow passageway. While in some cases an injury such as a fracture to the wrist, fluid retention or a build-up of fat within the carpal tunnel might cause this, in arthritis sufferers it is the swelling and inflammation of the lubricating membrane (the synovium) of the tendons which is the source of the problem. When this occurs, not only does it lead to pain in the palm side of the thumb, index finger, middle finger, the inside half of the ring finger and the hand, but also to numbness and tingling in these areas. As the median nerve also provides muscle power to the thumb, weakness in the thumb can also be experienced, which can make it difficult for sufferers to hold objects securely, and some complain of shooting pains from the hand right up to the shoulder.

Depending on the severity of the condition, sufferers may experience few or no symptoms during the day, and when these do occur they may only be brought on by certain activities such as typing, writing or doing housework. In other cases, however, they may be present throughout the day. Generally though, symptoms tend to be worse at night and many of those who suffer from carpal tunnel syndrome complain of disturbed sleep as a result.

Although in some cases surgery can help to relieve the pressure on the median nerve, because carpal tunnel syndrome caused by arthritis tends to come about due to inflammation of the membrane covering the tendons, an operation is not usually beneficial. A steroid injection into the wrist joint, however, can provide effective relief which lasts for several weeks, and sufferers can also benefit from the wearing of a splint at night or when carrying out the activities which typically aggravate their symptoms.

Depression and Anxiety

Depression and anxiety are two conditions which not only affect many sufferers of arthritis, but also those with a range of other chronic conditions. The shock of learning that they have a long-term illness which could potentially lead to serious complications or disability, or at the very least which might impair the individual's quality of life or require lifestyle adjustments can frequently lead to feelings of panic and worry, and eventually to those of utter despair and hopelessness.

Anxiety, which quite often develops as the result of a distressing event or situation such as being diagnosed with a chronic illness, can in itself be an insidious condition because anxiety breeds anxiety to the extent where the sufferer lives in a constant state of fear. What typically happens is that the initial anxious feelings start to lead to physical symptoms such as:

- Sweating
- Shaking
- Dizziness
- Hyperventilation
- Increased heartbeat
- Extreme tiredness
- Loss of appetite
- Insomnia
- Indigestion
- Unexplained aches and pains
- Diarrhoea

These symptoms then create the basis for further anxiety as the sufferer starts to imagine that they are the result of physiological illness. That is not to say that their physical symptoms are not real, because they most certainly are. They do not, however, arise from a physical cause, but rather an emotional or psychological one. In more severe cases, terrifying panic attacks can occur and some anxiety sufferers also experience symptoms of phobias, as well as exhibiting obsessive or compulsive behaviours.

Depression, which frequently goes hand in hand with anxiety, is not, as some people imagine, just about feeling a bit low and it is not something that sufferers can just snap out of. It is a potentially very serious medical condition which can not only affect an individual's ability to take pleasure in anything in life, but also their ability to function normally. In severe cases, it can lead sufferers into such despair that the only way out that they can see is by taking their own lives.

The symptoms of depression can be quite wide ranging, but some of the most common include:

- Feelings of despair and helplessness
- Low self-esteem
- Lack of interest in normal everyday activities and the things which previously gave pleasure
- Feelings of uselessness and inadequacy
- Lack of motivation
- Indecisiveness
- Irritability and intolerance
- Difficulties with concentration
- Extreme tiredness
- Insomnia
- Loss of appetite
- Unexplained aches and pains
- Slow movement and/or speech
- Social withdrawal and self-imposed isolation
- Suicidal thoughts

Depression and anxiety are both complex conditions and it is not understood why some people seem to be more prone to them than others. Because they both involve the emotions and the workings of the mind, sometimes they can be triggered quite unexpectedly through links with events or situations which happened long ago but which we might have buried somewhere deep inside our sub-conscious minds. Thus, being diagnosed with or living with a chronic illness might in itself cause a bout of anxiety or depression, but so might the association of the feelings experienced at this time with disturbing past events.

Although there are medications such as antidepressants and tranquilisers which can help in the short term for depression and anxiety, counselling and psychotherapy are typically much more effective because they provide sufferers with an understanding of the deeper underlying issues, as well as providing them with the tools for long-lasting recovery so that they are able to spot the early signs and know how to deal with them before the situation spirals out of control.

As you can imagine, the physical symptoms of depression and anxiety can add hugely to the existing symptoms caused by arthritis and other chronic pain conditions. The constant tensing of muscles which is typical when we feel stressed can aggravate existing pain, and symptoms such as headaches, insomnia and loss of appetite can all add to the arthritis patient's distress. Seeking treatment for depression or anxiety is therefore essential to help restore emotional, psychological and physical well-being.

Diabetes

Although arthritis and diabetes are two entirely different diseases which affect the body in very different ways, there do appear to be some interesting connections between them and a good deal of overlap. In fact, research conducted in more recent years has shown that people who have diabetes are almost twice as likely to suffer from arthritis.

Diabetes is a condition which affects the blood sugar levels in the body and there are two types of the disease. In Type 1, the beta cells in the pancreas which normally create and release insulin are destroyed by an autoimmune disease so that the body does not produce the hormone at all. As insulin is needed to carry glucose (a type of sugar) into the body's cells so that it can be converted into energy, without it, the levels of glucose in the blood build up and the body's cells sustain damage. In Type 2, the more common form of diabetes, the body does not use insulin properly (this is known as insulin resistance) and the beta cells gradually stop functioning so that less and less insulin is produced over time. Again, the result is that blood sugar levels rise and the body's cells become starved of energy and are damaged.

In the case of Type 1 diabetes it is essential for the insulin which is missing from the body to be replaced by using insulin injections, although patients also need to be extremely careful in terms of lifestyle choices such as those affecting diet and exercise. In earlier stages of Type 2 diabetes, meanwhile, lifestyle changes alone can sometimes be sufficient to control blood sugar levels, but often patients also need to take oral medication to keep these within safe and healthy limits. As the disease progresses, they may also need to rely on insulin injections. If diabetes remains untreated, there is a considerable risk that the high levels of glucose in the blood could cause nerve damage and damage to the large and small blood vessels. This in turn can lead to poor circulation, heart attacks, strokes, kidney disease or even kidney failure, as well as to damage to the eyes.

Although both types of diabetes can develop in people of any age, Type 1 tends to be first diagnosed in those under the age of 20, whereas Type 2 is more common in people over 40. In the UK, it is estimated that around 5% of those over the age of 65 and around 20% of those over 85 have Type 2 diabetes, but perhaps as many as one million others in the country have the disease but have not yet been diagnosed with it. The total number of individuals to have either Type 1 or Type 2 diabetes in the UK is thought to be around 2.8 million.

In the USA, meanwhile, almost 19 million people have been diagnosed with the illness, but a further 7 million are suspected to be undiagnosed. In addition, a massive 79 million people in America are believed to suffer from pre-diabetes, a state in which blood sugar levels are higher than they should be, but not high enough to indicate Type 2 diabetes. This condition is also sometimes referred to as impaired glucose tolerance and it may be the case that those who suffer from pre-diabetes are already suffering long-term damage to the heart and circulatory system in particular. If pre-diabetes is left untreated, it can develop into Type 2 diabetes, usually within less than 10 years.

As I have mentioned, Type 1 diabetes is believed to be an auto-immune disorder in which the body's own immune system attacks otherwise healthy cells. Type 2, however, which tends to run in families, is often closely linked to being overweight or obese. In addition, those in the following categories are also believed to be at greater risk:

- Those who have a parent, child, brother or sister with Type 2 diabetes
- People over 40
- People with sedentary lifestyles
- Women with a waist measurement of more than 31.5 inches and men whose waists measure more than 37 inches
- Women who suffered from Type 2 diabetes or impaired glucose tolerance during pregnancy
- People with pre-diabetes

Although the symptoms of Type 1 diabetes tend to develop quite quickly, usually over the course of days or weeks, those for Type 2 often appear more gradually. In either case, however, the most common signs of the disease include:

- Being very thirsty
- Frequent urination
- Tiredness
- Feeling very hungry
- Unusual weight loss
- Changes in the ability of the body to heal itself from cuts and sores
- Dryness or itchiness of the skin, particularly around the penis or vagina
- Recurring bouts of thrush
- Numbness or tingling sensations in the feet due to poor circulation or nerve damage
- Blurring of vision caused by the dryness of the lenses of the eyes

If diabetes goes untreated or if the sufferer is unwell or eats too much, then blood sugar levels can become very high, resulting in hyperglycaemia. The symptoms of hyperglycaemia are similar to the main ones experienced in diabetes, particularly thirst and dryness of the mouth, a frequent need to urinate, blurred vision and drowsiness, but often these are more severe or they come on more suddenly. If hyperglycaemia is not treated, it can lead to diabetic ketoacidosis, which can cause the sufferer to lose consciousness and is potentially life-threatening. In all cases, however, being diagnosed early with diabetes is extremely important so that the risk of developing complications is reduced.

As I have said, people who have diabetes are almost twice as likely to suffer from arthritis and, in the case of osteoarthritis, both age and excess body weight or obesity are two of the risk factors for both this and Type 2 diabetes. In addition, this type of diabetes seems to cause greater levels of inflammation in the body, which serves to aggravate the symptoms, not only of osteoarthritis, but also of the many other forms of the disease. Because diabetes can cause problems with nerves, the connective tissues and even the joints, sometimes joint pain, stiffness and swelling similar to that seen in various types of arthritic conditions can also develop in diabetics.

In Type 1 diabetes and rheumatoid arthritis in particular, studies have shown several similarities. First of all, sufferers of both conditions tend to have elevated levels of C-reactive protein and interleukin-6 (both proteins in the blood whose levels rise in response to inflammation). In addition, an increase in tumour necrosis factor-alpha (TNF-a), a chemical substance which delivers messages between the cells of the body and is also involved in the inflammatory process, has been shown to exist in those who have had Type 1 diabetes for more than five years, as well as those with inflammatory forms of arthritis. There may also be a genetic connection between Type 1 diabetes and rheumatoid arthritis, as well as between Type 1 and juvenile idiopathic arthritis, as researchers have identified a gene called PTPN22 which seems to be present in many sufferers of each of these diseases.

Interestingly, it is not only the levels of inflammatory markers and the presence of genes which are helping to establish links between diabetes and arthritis, but also arthritis treatments. Certain of the biologic agents which are used to treat inflammatory arthritis seem to improve insulin resistance and help to control glucose levels in those with Type 2 diabetes. On the negative side, however, the corticosteroids which are often used to treat the inflammation caused by arthritis have been shown to interfere with the way that glucose is metabolised in the body, and it is thought that this could lead to the development of Type 1 diabetes.

Although diabetes is not a cause of arthritis, or vice versa, as you can see, some of the risk factors for developing each of these conditions are shared, as are some of the symptoms. Perhaps more so than with other conditions, the links between arthritis and Type 2 diabetes illustrate the importance of a holistic approach to treatment and the need to look after our overall well-being.

Fibromyalgia

Fibromyalgia is a little understood but extremely common condition which is believed to affect hundreds of millions of people around the world. In the UK and the USA alone, it is estimated that between 2% and 4.5% of the population could be suffering from its effects, although these statistics are hard to verify because so many cases are believed to go unreported. Irrespective of where in the world sufferers live or originate from, a massive 80–90% are women, with those between the ages of 40 and 55 appearing to be at greater risk. The condition does appear in men too, however, as well as in children and the elderly, but in the vast majority of cases, onset is seen in middle-aged women who are approaching or have reached menopause.

Although the aches, pains and stiffness which are characteristic of fibromyalgia often feel as though they are coming from the joints, this is in fact a condition in which widespread and extreme pain affects any of a number of different muscle groups around the body. Often it is the neck, back, shoulders, pelvic region and the hands which are most severely affected, but as you can see from Figure 4.2, there are 18 specific 'tender points' which doctors take into consideration when making their diagnosis of fibromyalgia. These 'tender points' are areas of soft tissue which, if subjected to even the slightest pressure, generate various levels of pain which might be deep and aching or shooting, burning, gnawing or radiating.

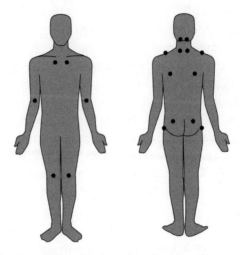

Figure 4.2 The 18 'tender points' used to diagnose fibromyalgia

The symptoms of fibromyalgia are not just restricted to pain, however, and many sufferers experience:

- Stiffness
- Numbness and tingling sensations
- Muscle spasms
- Cramps
- Chronic fatigue
- Sleep disorders, and
- Cognitive and memory impairment

In addition, the condition is commonly linked with:

- Headaches
- Migraines
- Irritable bowel syndrome
- Temporomandibular joint dysfunction (TMJD)
- Painful bladder syndrome (interstitial cystitis)
- Premenstrual syndrome (PMS)

- Intolerance to heat or cold
- Restless leg syndrome
- Periodic limb movement disorder, and
- Depression and anxiety

So diverse are the symptoms of fibromyalgia, in fact, that there are still those in the medical fraternity who do not accept the condition as being a real physical complaint, believing it instead to be all in the mind. Their scepticism is not helped by the fact that fibromyalgia appears to cause no distinguishable physiological damage to the body. As I have seen in treating thousands of suffers of this condition, however, and as anyone who is diagnosed with fibromyalgia will attest to, not only does it cause extreme pain and suffering in many cases, but it also has the potential to have a devastating impact on the quality of the sufferer's life.

Although the precise cause of fibromyalgia has not been identified, a number of theories abound. While some credit the condition to a dysfunction of the central nervous system, chemical or hormonal imbalances, genetic factors, a disorder of the immune system, environmental factors, infections, and even directly to sleep disorders, others attribute it to physical traumas and injuries. In the latter case, it is notable that many of those who develop fibromyalgia do so in the wake of an accident in which they sustained a whiplash-type injury.

Because fibromyalgia does not cause any discernible changes or damage to the muscles, ligaments or tendons of the body and because it does not directly affect the joints, it cannot therefore be considered a form of arthritis, and in fact has been categorically ruled out as such. Having said this, however, fibromyalgia and many forms of arthritis can be very difficult to diagnose without any single blood or other type of test to identify their presence, which can cause difficulties for those doctors who are not particularly well-acquainted with or experienced in them. Not only is there sometimes confusion between fibromyalgia and arthritis, but also between fibromyalgia and a variety of other conditions, including chronic fatigue syndrome, myofascial pain syndrome, Gulf War syndrome and Lyme disease.

Despite the fact that in many ways fibromyalgia and arthritis are very different conditions, because they are both chronic diseases, they do have the potential to affect sufferers' lives in similar ways. In both cases, not only are there physical repercussions, but also emotional and psychological ones too, all of which can have severe implications on quality of life. With a multidisciplinary approach to treatment, however, there is much that can be done to alleviate pain and to successfully manage each of these conditions so that any impact is minimised.

Osteoporosis

One of the main reasons why there is often confusion between osteoporosis and arthritis is simply because of the similarity between the name of the former and the most common form of arthritis, osteoarthritis. Although 'osteo' in both cases means 'bone', in osteoarthritis it is the ends of the bone within the joint capsule which are affected, whereas in osteoporosis it could be any part of the bone. As can be seen from Figure 4.3, in the latter case the bones become less dense and more porous, making them weaker, more brittle and much more likely to fracture.

Normal bone   Bone with osteoporosis

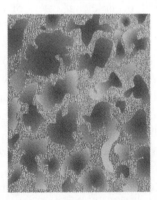

Figure 4.3 The effects of osteoporosis

Osteoporosis is believed to affect around 3 million people in the UK and 10 million in the USA, although statistics vary considerably from one source to another, mainly because the condition often goes undiagnosed until a fracture actually occurs. The disease, however, is reported to account for 240,000 fractures each year in the UK and around 1.5 million in the USA, and some sources estimate that 50% of women and 20% of men over the age of 50 will incur a fracture as a result of the condition. Like many forms of arthritis, osteoporosis is a disease which primarily affects women, and particularly those who are postmenopausal.

Although many people tend to think of bone as being formed before we are born, growing throughout childhood and adolescence and then remaining the same throughout the rest of our lives, it does in fact continually undergo a process of constant renewal. At the same time as old bone is being broken down by cells known as osteoclasts, new bone is being produced by osteoblasts, but the speed at which these two things happen changes as we grow older. When we are children, our bodies form new bone very quickly so that our bones grow in length, whereas during adolescence and in our early 20s, they stop becoming longer but grow stronger and denser, reaching their maximum density by the time we are in our mid-20s. Between the ages of around 25–40, there is then a stable period during which the rate at which older bone is broken down and new bone is produced is about equal. From 40 onwards, however, the balance shifts and older bone starts to be broken down more quickly than new bone is produced, leading to a gradual loss of bone density. Although this is a process which happens in all of us, only when bone mass falls below certain levels would a person be diagnosed with osteoporosis.

There are two significant reasons why women are at greater risk of osteoporosis than men. First of all, in the run-up to their 40s, men generally reach a higher level of bone density than women, so that in effect, when the process of bone loss does start to occur, they have a head start. In addition, however, when women's bodies stop producing the hormone oestrogen, there is a period of several years after menopause during which the process of bone loss speeds up, causing levels of bone density to fall dangerously low.

Growing older and being female though, are not the only two risk factors for osteoporosis and a number of other things can affect the likelihood of males and females of younger ages developing the condition, including:

■ Oestrogen deficiency – women who have a hysterectomy, who have one or both ovaries removed or who naturally go into menopause before the age of 45 stop producing oestrogen earlier and so their bodies become deficient in the hormone

■ A sedentary lifestyle – exercise helps to keep the bones strong and healthy, but in those whose lifestyles are more sedentary there is a greater loss of calcium which causes the bones to become weaker and increases the chances of developing osteoporosis

■ Poor diet – calcium and vitamin D (which helps the body to absorb calcium) are both essential for maintaining strong bones, so a diet which is deficient in these elements, whether due to eating disorders or any other reason, makes the condition more likely

■ Being thin or small-framed – people who are naturally thinner or small-framed have smaller or thinner bones so there is less bone density to lose

■ Smoking – both male and female sex hormones are relevant in terms of bone density and as smoking affects the levels of these hormones, not only are female smokers at greater risk of osteoporosis due to reduced levels of oestrogen, but male smokers are more likely to develop the disease because of low levels of testosterone

■ High alcohol consumption – alcohol affects the ability of the body's cells to produce new bone, so that the balance of degeneration and regeneration is unfavourably altered

■ A family history of the condition – osteoporosis does seem to run in families, so anyone who has a close family relative who suffers from the disease is at greater risk

Another very important group of people who are at greater risk of osteoporosis but which I have not mentioned so far is those who use corticosteroid medications, and this is where one of the main links between this condition and arthritis comes in. Corticosteroids are one of the main drugs to be used in the treatment of inflammatory types of arthritis, particularly rheumatoid arthritis, and because these medications can reduce the amount of calcium which is absorbed into the body, they can cause bones to become weakened and increase the chances of developing osteoporosis. In fact, this is one of the main reasons why doctors will normally try to reduce the dosages of corticosteroids as quickly as possible after treatment for arthritis has begun. In addition to this, however, the inflammatory process which is typical in conditions like rheumatoid arthritis can in itself also lead to the loss of bone density.

Despite the fact that some forms of arthritis can directly or indirectly lead to osteoporosis though, the symptoms of the conditions are quite different. Whereas in arthritis pain and swelling of the joints are two of the most common signs, in the case of osteoporosis there are often no symptoms at all and the sufferer does not even know of their condition until a bone fracture is incurred. In most cases, this happens as the result of only a minor fall or accident, but even coughing or sneezing has been known to cause bones to break.

The bones which tend to be at greatest risk in osteoporosis are the hips, wrists and spine, and where the latter is involved, the damage to the vertebrae can lead to a decrease in height, as well as curvature of the spine and the characteristic 'dowager's hump'. In more severe cases, the reduced amount of space under the ribs caused by compression of the spine or changes to its shape can also lead to breathing difficulties.

Osteoporosis can be a very serious condition and there is an estimated 10–20% mortality rate within six months in those who sustain fractures of the hip. Of the remainder, as many as 50% may be unable to walk without assistance and a further 25% are likely to require long-term care. Minor fractures, on the other hand, tend to heal quite successfully on their own and in many cases do not cause considerable amounts of pain. As is the case with arthritis, however, there are many excellent treatments available to help sufferers of osteoporosis and much that they can do in terms of exercise, diet and lifestyle changes to improve their condition and their overall quality of life.

Paget's Disease of the Bone

Paget's disease of the bone, or osteitis deformans, is a disease which can lead to the most common form of arthritis, namely osteoarthritis. It is quite distinct from, and bears no relation to Paget's disease of the breast, which is a rare form of breast cancer. For ease, however, I will refer to Paget's disease of the bone simply as Paget's disease throughout the remainder of this book.

After osteoporosis, Paget's disease is the most common disease of the bone and for some unknown reason it is most prevalent in the UK, although those countries which have experienced an influx of people of British descent over the years, such as the USA, Australia, New Zealand and South Africa, also tend to see more cases than elsewhere. The condition rarely affects people below the age of 40, but it is estimated that 2–3% of those over 50 in the UK have the condition, with the chances of it developing increasing with age. Men suffer from Paget's disease more often than women, with around 8% of men and 5% of women being affected.

As I described under the heading of osteoporosis, bone is constantly being renewed by cells called osteoclasts and osteoblasts, but in Paget's disease this process is very much speeded up, to the extent that the rate of bone turnover can be increased by up to as much as 40 times. Not only does this cause the size of bones to be increased, possibly causing deformity and causing nerves to become compressed, but as can be seen from Figure 4.4, when new bone is generated, its shape and structure is irregular and weaker than normal, compact bone so that the risk of fracture is increased. Both the compression of nerves in the skull and the thickening of the bones around the ears can cause hearing loss and even total deafness in sufferers of Paget's disease.

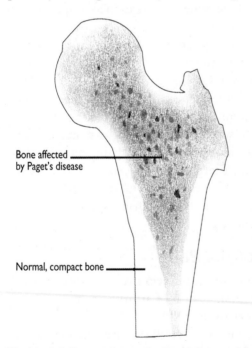

Bone affected by Paget's disease

Normal, compact bone

Figure 4.4 Comparison of normal bone with bone affected by Paget's disease

The bones most commonly affected by Paget's disease are those in the thighs and shins, the pelvis, the spine and the skull, but the disease is not always painful and is sometimes only diagnosed when the patient has blood tests or X-rays taken as part of the diagnosis or ongoing monitoring of other conditions. Where symptoms are experienced, pain in the bone itself is the most common, but where the disease works its way to the ends of the bones, then osteoarthritis can develop with its characteristic joint pain and stiffness. Although only in rare cases, Paget's disease can sometimes lead to the development of benign or malignant tumours in the bone which typically cause increased pain and swelling.

Although most patients also require the help of pain-killing medications, the treatment of Paget's disease is largely focussed on slowing down the rate of bone turnover through the use of bisphosphonates, a group of drugs which helps to prevent the loss of bone mass by working chiefly on the cells which are responsible for breaking down old bone. Ensuring a diet which is sufficient in calcium and vitamin D is also important for sufferers of the condition.

Sjögren's Syndrome

As we saw in Chapter 3, Sjögren's syndrome is frequently associated with several different types of arthritis, namely polymyositis and dermatomyositis, scleroderma, systemic lupus erythematosus and rheumatoid arthritis, all of which are believed to be autoimmune disorders. The condition does not, however, only appear in conjunction with other illnesses, but also as an autoimmune disorder in its own right.

Sjögren's syndrome is thought to affect around half a million people in the UK, but because many people never consult a doctor about their symptoms this figure could be wildly inaccurate. Approximately 90% of sufferers are believed to be women between the ages of 40 and 60, but men and occasionally children can be affected by it too. It is not known why the immune system is caused to react in the way that it does in this condition, but there have been unsubstantiated claims that it could be triggered by certain types of virus.

Mainly it is the tear and salivary glands which are affected in Sjögren's syndrome. Antibodies attack the tissues and nerve signals to these glands, so that the amount of saliva and tears produced is reduced, leading to dry eyes and mouth. The eyes may also become sore and reddened or sticky with mucus and it is not uncommon for sufferers to find strong light to be uncomfortable. Symptoms affecting the mouth, meanwhile, frequently include mouth ulcers and difficulties with swallowing, and some complain of an altered sense of taste. Fungal infections of the mouth can occur too and the salivary glands may become painful. There may also be hoarseness or weakness of the voice or a dry cough.

The symptoms of Sjögren's syndrome, however, are not necessarily just confined to the eyes and mouth. Chronic fatigue is common amongst sufferers, as are pain and inflammation in the joints, which may be characterised by a general feeling of achiness or specific tender points around the body. In addition, the disorder is also associated with:

- Dryness and itchiness of the skin
- Sensitivity to strong sunlight
- Raynaud's syndrome, in which the hands and/or feet become very cold and turn from white to blue to red
- Headaches which feel similar to migraines
- Irritable bowel syndrome
- Pain in the lower abdomen
- Swollen lymph nodes in the neck, armpits and groin
- Numbness and weakness caused by problems with the nervous system
- Vasculitis, in which the blood vessels become inflamed
- Severe menopausal symptoms
- Inflammation of the lining of the lungs and chest, which is known as pleurisy
- Kidney or liver problems

The range of symptoms experienced by individual sufferers of Sjögren's syndrome can vary greatly, as can their severity, but there are many treatments available which can help to alleviate or improve these. Although a few people with the disorder do suffer pain and inflammation of the joints, usually this does not cause any additional damage above and beyond that which may be caused if the person also has arthritis.

Vasculitis

Vasculitis is a condition in which the blood vessels become inflamed and it can either occur on its own or secondary to other diseases and disorders, of which rheumatoid arthritis, systemic lupus erythematosus, polymyalgia rheumatica and dermatomyositis are just a few. There are a number of different types of the condition which tend to affect different groups of people of different ages and genders, including:

- Takayasu's arteritis
- Kawasaki disease
- Behcet's disease
- Buerger's disease
- Wegener's granulomatosis
- Churg-Strauss syndrome
- Henoch-Schönlein purpura
- Polyarteritis nodosa (PAN)
- Microscopic polyangiitis
- Hypersensitivity vasculitis
- Cryoglobulin-associated vasculitis, and
- Temporal arteritis, which is also known as giant cell arteritis

Around 3,000 new cases of the different forms of vasculitis are reported in the UK each year, but the symptoms of the condition and the consequential damage to the blood vessels and the body's tissues and organs can vary enormously depending upon which blood vessels are affected and to what extent.

As you can see from Figure 4.5, the inflammation caused by vasculitis can lead to several different outcomes. In some cases, as the walls of the blood vessel swell due to inflammation, this causes a narrowing of the vessel which restricts the flow of blood or even an occlusion or sudden blocking of the vessel. In other cases, the blood vessel walls can become so stretched and weakened that they begin to bulge in what is known as an aneurysm and should the vessel burst this of course leads to internal bleeding which in some cases can be very serious. In cases where the large blood vessels are involved or where the vessels feed organs such as the heart, lungs and kidneys, the damage is likely to be more substantial.

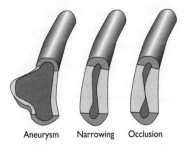

Aneurysm   Narrowing   Occlusion

Figure 4.5 Areaof inflammation on a blood vessel lining

Although there are often no outward signs of vasculitis, where the condition affects the skin, rashes of spots appear and these can sometimes rupture causing skin ulcers. Usually though, the patient tends to feel generally unwell and experiences:

- Fever
- Sweating
- Fatigue
- General aches and pains
- Loss of appetite
- Weight loss

Where other parts of the body are affected, however, this can lead to a variety of other symptoms, including:

- Inflammation of the nerves, causing tingling or weakness
- Shortness of breath, coughing and even coughing up blood where the lungs are affected
- Mouth ulcers or abdominal pain in cases where the gastrointestinal tract is affected
- Sinus problems, ear infections, ulcers in the nose and hearing loss

- Redness, itchiness and burning of the eyes, as well as sensitivity to light and blurred vision. In rare cases, blindness can also occur
- Headaches, inability to think clearly, changes in mental function, muscle weakness or paralysis where the brain is affected
- Difficulties in passing urine or blood in the urine where the kidneys are affected

Vasculitis which affects the kidneys can be quite dangerous because often the symptoms do not appear until the organs have already sustained damage.

As I mentioned earlier under the heading of Polymyalgia Rheumatica, around 20% of people with this particular form of arthritis will develop the form of vasculitis known as temporal or giant cell arteritis and 40–60% of those with the latter will also have symptoms of polymyalgia rheumatica. Should symptoms such as severe headaches, pain or swelling in the scalp, jaw pain, tenderness around the area of the temples or blurred or double vision appear, then urgent medical treatment should be sought as this type of vasculitis can cause blindness.

Although the treatment of vasculitis will depend on which form of the disease is diagnosed, corticosteroids are often the mainstay as these are generally very effective at reducing inflammation in the body. Different types of vasculitis, however, may require the prescription of other types of medication such as immunosuppressants or anti-bacterial drugs to control the disease and limit any potential damage to the tissues and organs. As smoking causes the blood vessels to constrict and so can make the symptoms of the disease worse, smokers will be advised to quit.

What Causes Arthritis?

As you will have seen from Chapter 3, although there are one or two notable exceptions, the most prevalent and most serious forms of arthritis, including osteoarthritis, rheumatoid arthritis, polymyalgia rheumatica, polymyositis and dermatomyositis, scleroderma and systemic lupus erythematosus (SLE) are all conditions which affect far greater numbers of women than men. Although there are almost certainly other factors which can increase the likelihood of suffering from one of these diseases, the link with hormones is not one which can be ignored and indeed ongoing research into arthritis not only seeks to discover the underlying causes, but also to develop gender-specific treatments.

The Hormone Theories

The three main types of sex hormone, namely oestrogen, progesterone and testosterone all exist in both males and females, although women normally have more oestrogen and progesterone and men normally have more testosterone. In terms of autoimmune disorders in particular, the hormone oestrogen is suspected to play a role in their development, but precisely what that role might be is not yet understood. Logically, if high concentrations of the hormone were to cause autoimmune diseases, then it would be reasonable to see the conditions of pregnant women with these disorders become worse, because of course oestrogen levels rise during pregnancy. Interestingly though, while many women who suffer from rheumatoid arthritis go into remission during pregnancy, those with SLE tend to get very much worse.

The way that oestrogen is metabolised in the body may provide some clues in terms of SLE. Depending upon diet and other environmental factors, the hormone can be broken down into feminising compounds which affect things like bone growth and blood clotting, as well as moods, behaviour and overall feelings of well-being, and non-feminising compounds. In both male and female sufferers of SLE, a number of very feminising compounds have been found to exist, and although scientists do not believe that these constitute an actual cause of the disease, they do suspect that it might set up a predisposition to it.

Research into the effects of testosterone, which is normally a protective substance in men, meanwhile, has also proved to be somewhat confusing. While men who have low levels of the hormone do seem to be at greater risk of all types of autoimmune diseases and an estimated one-third of men with autoimmune disorders have low levels of testosterone, because the other two-thirds show normal levels, this cannot be the actual cause of the conditions. In women with SLE, however, their bodies metabolise the hormone so quickly that their levels of testosterone are practically non-existent. Even though the male sex hormone seems to play a key role in the development of lupus, tests which involved boosting testosterone levels in female SLE patients showed that it did not bring about any improvement.

The Chromosome Theory

Another area that scientists are considering in relation to differences between the autoimmune responses of men and women is chromosomes. Men, of course, have an X and a Y chromosome, while women have two Xs, but in each cell of a woman's body, one of the X chromosomes is effectively switched off so that women do not have twice as many as men. Which one is switched off, however, is purely down to chance, but once it has been inactivated it stays that way. One school of thought is that the pattern in which X chromosomes are inactivated or an imbalance in this inactivation may be responsible for women having a higher risk of developing autoimmune disorders.

Killer Cells

Both male and female bodies play host to killer cells known as T cells and these too provide clues as to why men's immune systems may respond differently to women's. T cells are a type of white blood cell which circulates around our bodies and they are known as such because they mature in an organ in the chest called the thymus. Their job is to identify, attack and destroy viruses, infections and other invaders which enter the system and so they play a key role in the body's immune system.

Healthy men, however, have higher levels of T cells than healthy women do, which means that their bodies are very good at heading off invaders at the pass and stopping them before they have a chance to do any real harm. Women's bodies, on the other hand, do not have such good advanced warning systems and so their immune system responses are slightly delayed and are more likely to be caught off guard initially. When this does happen, because a woman's immune system is in fact incredibly robust, her body responds fiercely to the invaders, but of course in autoimmune diseases it is healthy cells and tissues which are attacked rather than unhealthy ones. The very fact that women's immune systems are so good at fighting back actually works against them in the case of autoimmunity, and would account for why they experience more severe symptoms in diseases such as rheumatoid arthritis.

Various studies have shown a low incidence of autoimmune diseases such as rheumatoid arthritis in men who have high levels of T cells in their bodies, and researchers are also finding that people of either sex who have reduced numbers of killer cells may be more likely to develop such disorders.

Male v Female Body Structures

Male and female bodies are built differently, and in more than just the obvious ways. In terms of how these differences might contribute to the most common form of arthritis, osteoarthritis, there are several factors which might be relevant and again, researchers are taking these into consideration in the development of gender-specific treatments.

As we saw in Chapter 3, osteoarthritis is far more common in women than in men and some sources estimate that women are twice as likely to develop osteoarthritis of the knee as their male counterparts. Three of the main anatomical differences which might account for this are:

- The knees in males and females are stabilised by different muscles. In women, it is the weaker quadriceps muscles at the fronts of the thighs which perform this task, whereas in men, it is the job of the stronger hamstrings at the backs of the thighs
- A woman's pelvis tips forward for reasons of childbearing which changes the angles of the bones and makes women more prone to hyperextending their knees (moving them beyond their normal range of motion). As the quadriceps muscles do not have enough power to stabilise the knees sufficiently, this may lead to joint damage
- Men have significantly more knee cartilage than women, simply because they are larger, which provides them with more natural protection

Even in the fittest and strongest of women, these basic anatomical differences still appear to put them at a disadvantage in terms of experiencing stress to the knees and of increasing their chances of developing osteoarthritis.

According to research undertaken in Australia and the USA, damage to one of the ligaments in the knee joint, the anterior cruciate ligament, leads to a greater likelihood of developing osteoarthritis and women sustain this type of damage more frequently than men, even through simple twists or falls. At one time, this was believed to be due to the hormonal fluctuations which take place during the menstrual cycle, but a more recent study has shown this theory to be unfounded. In fact, women are no more likely to sustain a rupture or tear to the lateral cruciate ligament than men, irrespective of where they are in their menstrual cycle or whether they are ingesting hormones through the use of contraceptives.

Having said this, however, post-menopausal women who have the lowest levels of oestrogen in their bodies are undoubtedly at greater risk of developing osteoarthritis of the knee. As I explained earlier in this chapter rather than the levels of the hormone in both males and females being responsible for the increased risk, it is suspected that the way in which oestrogen is metabolised in the body could be more significant.

Clearly there is still a long way to go before the underlying causes of arthritis are definitively identified, but in the meantime significant research is being undertaken on an ongoing basis to discover what triggers the different types of disease to develop and to allow scientists to develop a cure.

Diagnosing Arthritis

As you will have been able to see from Chapters 3 and 4, the many different types of arthritis, along with the assorted conditions which are frequently associated with the disease and those which present in similar ways, can sometimes make the job of diagnosing arthritis quite difficult. In addition, in some cases the symptoms can start and develop slowly and gradually and so the nature of the illness may take time to become fully evident. Patients, however, can do much to help those in the medical profession to arrive at a quick and accurate diagnosis by being able to offer an accurate description of their symptoms and a full account of their medical history and by knowing what to expect. Not only does this help doctors though, as in understanding the types of investigations that physicians may need to undertake patients can also save themselves a great deal of worry or fear.

Questions to Expect

The first things that the doctor will need to understand when you visit are the symptoms or problems which have led you to seek medical attention and any factors relating to your past medical history which might be relevant. Sometimes patients find it helpful to keep a diary of their symptoms or to write down what they can remember in advance of their visit so as not to miss anything out at a time when they might be feeling quite nervous. Some of the questions that you are likely to be asked include:

- What are the main symptoms or problems that you are experiencing?
- Have you experienced any other symptoms?

- How long have you had the symptoms?
- When and how did they begin?
- Where precisely does it hurt?
- Are there certain times when the symptoms feel worse? E.g. After certain activities or periods of inactivity
- Is there anything that makes the symptoms worse or better?
- Can you describe the pain? I.e. Is it dull or sharp, achy, burning or grinding?
- Do your symptoms come and go or are they there constantly?
- How long does the pain usually last?
- Overall, have your symptoms got worse, better or stayed the same since they first began?
- Have you experienced any swelling or redness in any of your joints?
- Do you experience stiffness in any of your joints?
- Do you experience the symptoms on just one side of your body or both?
- Do your symptoms affect your ability to carry out your daily tasks or your work?
- Do you have any other medical conditions?
- Have you recently sustained an injury to the affected joint?
- Have you recently overused the affected joint?
- Have you recently suffered from any type of infection?
- Do any of your family members suffer from similar problems or symptoms?
- Have any of your relatives ever been diagnosed with arthritis?
- Are you currently taking any forms of medication? If so, what dosage are you on and how frequently do you take the medication?
- Do you have any allergies?
- Have you recently undergone any type of surgery or other medical procedure?

If your doctor suspects a particular type of arthritis, such as gout or rheumatoid arthritis, there may be additional questions that he or she will need to ask and it is important to be prepared for these too, not least so that you do not take offence at his or her reason for asking. In the case of gout, for example, you may be asked about your alcohol intake or your diet or the use of certain drugs such as water tablets. As we have seen, certain other types of arthritis, meanwhile, are more likely in intravenous drug users or those at risk of sexually transmitted infections, so if the doctor does enquire about these issues it is because he or she needs to rule in or out these possibilities. It is vital that you answer these and any other questions honestly and fully to help your doctor make an accurate diagnosis and prescribe the most appropriate treatment programme.

Another important thing to remember is that if you have already visited other physicians in relation to your current condition, try to obtain any X-rays or reports which were produced at the time and take these along with you at the time of your appointment.

Physical Examinations

Having discussed your symptoms and medical history with you, your doctor will then need to carry out a physical examination to look for visible signs of the condition. Depending upon the type of arthritis that the doctor suspects, the sort of signs that he or she may look for could include:

- Tenderness
- Swelling
- Warmth
- Redness
- Pain on movement
- Stiffness or loss of movement in the joints
- Damage caused by bony growths in or around the joint
- Joint deformities
- The number of joints affected
- The pattern of affected joints
- Rashes or markings on the face or body
- Evidence of rheumatoid nodules under the skin
- Evidence of calcium deposits or tophi under the skin if pseudogout or gout is suspected

The doctor may ask you to stand up and carry out certain movements during the examination to assess how your range of motion and mobility have been affected.

Diagnostic Tests

As we saw in Chapter 3, there is a whole range of tests that your doctor may decide to carry out in his or her bid to diagnose your condition. Because there is no single, definitive test which will indicate the presence of arthritis or the type of the disease, some of these are aimed directly at spotting characteristic evidence, while others are used to rule out other conditions with similar symptoms. To follow, you will find a summary of the main types of test used to help diagnose some of the different forms of arthritis.

Blood Tests

Although blood tests are not usually a definitive diagnostic tool when they are considered alone, when their results are evaluated alongside the pattern of symptoms, the patient's medical history and a physical examination, they can often give the doctor significant clues. They can, for example, determine:

- The presence of inflammation in the body by checking the levels of different proteins, such as in erythrocyte sedimentation rate (ESR) and C-reactive protein (CRP) tests
- The presence of infection or inflammation via blood counts
- The presence of rheumatoid factor, an antibody which is found in the majority of cases of rheumatoid arthritis and other autoimmune conditions
- The presence of the *HLA-B27* gene which might indicate, for example, ankylosing spondylitis or reactive or psoriatic arthritis
- The presence of abnormal antibodies such as those found in autoimmune disorders through anti-nuclear antibody (ANA) tests. Other antibody tests can also be used to detect fungal or other types of infection
- The levels of iron, calcium and copper in the blood which might indicate certain other conditions such as haemochromatosis, hyperparathyroidism and Wilson's disease
- Uric acid levels where gout is suspected
- Calcium levels where pseudogout is suspected
- Decreased levels of proteins via a serum complement level test where an autoimmune disease is suspected

Urine Tests

Just like blood tests, urine tests can also help doctors to rule in or out certain arthritic or other types of conditions, although again they can only give indications rather than offering a definitive diagnosis. They can also be extremely useful in checking whether internal organs such as the liver or kidneys have been affected by systemic illness. Some of the most common urine tests are used to check the presence of:

- White blood cells and nitrites, both of which usually indicate an infection in the body
- Red blood cells, which may suggest bleeding in the urinary tract or infection
- Glucose, which may point to diabetes
- Ketones, which are normally only present in diabetes or eating disorders
- Protein, which usually only shows up where kidney disease or diabetes is present

X-rays

An X-ray is essentially a form of electromagnetic radiation which is similar to light. When an X-ray machine is used in a medical setting it basically sends out individual X-ray particles called photons which pass through the body. A special film or computer is then used to record the images which are created, and depending upon the structures that the photons have encountered on their journey, those images will show areas of white, black or grey. Dense structures such as bone, as well as metal and special dyes which are used to highlight areas of the body, for example, block out most of the photons and so show up as white, while structures containing air are black. Anything such as muscle, fat or fluid, meanwhile, will appear as a shade of grey.

X-rays can not only help to detect the signs of arthritis, but are also useful in ruling out things like fractures and other types of injuries, and even tumours. By allowing doctors to see the structures of the joints, they can alert him or her to damage to cartilage and bone, bony overgrowths and areas of calcification and infection, any of which may be characteristic of certain types of arthritis. X-rays which are taken for diagnostic purposes and then repeated during the course of treatment can also show doctors whether the treatment is having beneficial effects and/or slowing down the progress of the disease.

X-rays are performed in a radiology department, are completely painless and usually take no more than 10–15 minutes in total to carry out.

MRI Scans

Magnetic resonance imaging or MRI scans use magnetic and radio waves to create very clear images on a computer screen and are particularly useful for looking at the soft tissues in and around the joints, such as the muscles, ligaments, tendons and nerves, although they can see bone too. They are much more expensive for doctors to carry out than X-rays, but many believe that they carry the advantage of being able to detect damage sooner and so allow treatment to begin earlier.

Carrying out an MRI scan usually takes between 40 and 80 minutes, during which time the patient will normally be asked to wear a hospital gown and will then be placed on a sliding table. Older models of MRI scanners are normally enclosed and so the patient will effectively be inside a round tunnel when the images are taken, whereas new models are open. As the scanner captures the pictures of the affected area of the body, these are monitored by a technician and recorded so that they can be analysed by the doctor and help him or her to make a diagnosis. In some cases, patients may need to be injected with a special dye to help make the images clearer and in all cases it is necessary to keep as still as possible as movement causes the images to be less clear.

The process of capturing images using an MRI scan is in no way painful and in fact what most patients notice more than anything is the sound of the machine, which some have compared with what it must sound like to be inside a washing machine.

Joint Aspiration

The medical term for joint aspiration is arthrocentesis and, as explained in Chapter 3, the process involves using a sterilised hollow needle and syringe to drain some of the synovial fluid from within the joint capsule. Once the fluid has been collected, the subsequent analysis can then help doctors to identify any signs of infection and to decide which particular type of arthritis the patient might be suffering from. The presence of a fungal infection, for example, tells the doctor that fungal arthritis is the problem, while the presence of uric acid or calcium crystals suggests gout or pseudogout respectively.

As well as being used to help diagnose arthritis, joint aspiration is also used in certain cases as part of a treatment programme. Where an excess of synovial fluid has built up in a joint and is causing swelling, this can be drained off to relieve discomfort. If the fluid contains white blood cells which are actively destroying the joint, then arthrocentesis will not only help to preserve it, but also to alleviate inflammation and pain. In some cases, joint aspiration may be followed by injection of medication into the joint.

When arthrocentesis is carried out, the skin over the joint is sterilised before local anaesthetic is given in the form of an injection or by freezing the skin. Most people describe the procedure as being nothing more than mildly uncomfortable.

Synovial Biopsy

Although not regularly used to diagnose arthritis, a synovial biopsy can prove to be particularly useful in the diagnosis of gout, pseudogout, fungal and rheumatoid arthritis, as well as to check for the presence of bacterial infections. The procedure is carried out under local anaesthetic and involves taking a small sample of the synovial membrane which lines the affected joint for analysis.

Once the local anaesthetic has been injected into the area, a sharply pointed instrument called a trocar is inserted into the joint space and then a biopsy needle is pushed through the trocar and used to extract the sample. The biopsy site is then cleaned and pressure applied, after which the area is dressed with a bandage. The injection of the anaesthetic is typically felt as a prick and then a slight burning sensation and the insertion of the trocar may cause some discomfort.

Muscle Biopsy

A muscle biopsy can be particularly useful in the diagnosis of poly-myositis and dermatomyositis and involves taking a small sample of muscle to check for chronic inflammation and muscle degeneration and regeneration. As discussed earlier, ideally the sample needs to be taken from a muscle which is currently showing weakness and in which inflammation has been detected by an MRI scan.

One of two procedures might be used to perform a muscle biopsy, but in either case it is likely to be done under local rather than general anaesthetic. In the first, a hollow biopsy needle is used to pull out a small sample of muscle tissue, whereas in the second a small incision is made to expose the muscle, the sample is taken and then the wound is closed up using self-dissolving stitches on the inside and non-soluble stitches on the surface of the skin. In most cases the patient is able to return home later the same day, but sometimes an overnight stay is advisable if the latter technique is used. Where an incision does need to be made, the patient should avoid using the affected area of the body for the first day and should keep the wound dry for the first few days. It is usually necessary to avoid any undue exertion to the affected area for a couple of weeks after the operation.

Athroscopy

Arthroscopy is a technique which is either used to take a look inside a joint or to repair any damage that might have occurred. It is a form of keyhole surgery which, when used for diagnostic purposes, usually only involves making a single small incision and inserting an arthroscope (a flexible tube which is roughly the length and dia-meter of a drinking straw) into the joint. The arthroscope has a light and a camera on its tip and the images of the inside of the joint are transmitted onto a screen, giving the doctor a clear view and allowing him or her to assess the problem. When the procedure is complete, the site of the incision will be closed up with stitches and bandaged. Depending on which joint is involved and how long the arthroscopy is likely to take, it might be carried out under local, regional or general anaesthetic.

Where arthroscopy is used to carry out a surgical procedure such as repairing damaged ligaments or tendons, or removing loose bone or cartilage, the surgeon would make two or more incisions, one through which to insert the arthroscope and one or more through which to insert the other surgical instruments that he or she needs to use. Synovial biopsies are sometimes carried out using arthroscopy instead of a biopsy needle.

Electromyography (EMG) Test

An EMG test is a technique which is used to assess and record the electrical activity produced by the muscles and to check the health of the muscles themselves, as well as the nerves that control them. Although it is not helpful in the diagnosis of many types of arthritis, it can be particularly useful in identifying abnormal patterns of electrical activity in those suspected to be suffering from polymyositis or dermatomyositis.

In order to carry out the test, the doctor needs to insert a very fine needle electrode through the skin and into the muscle, which may feel slightly uncomfortable and similar to having an injection. The electrode then picks up the electrical activity from the muscle and the signal is sent to a receiver and the results displayed on a computer screen. You may be asked to contract the muscle during the course of the test so that the doctor can see how well your muscle responds when the nerve stimulates it to move.

Other Tests

Particularly where one of the systemic forms of arthritis is suspected, doctors may choose to carry out various other tests to check whether other parts of the body or internal organs have been affected. These might, for example, include heart scans, skin biopsies or tests to check lung functions.

Questions to Ask

Although your doctor may not be able to diagnose your condition definitively until after various tests have been completed and he or she is in receipt of the results, when you are informed of the diagnosis, it is important that you fill in any gaps in your knowledge and understanding while you have the opportunity. Often it helps to have these prepared and written down before the visit so that nothing is overlooked. You will almost certainly want to know, for example:

- Whether you do in fact have arthritis and, if so, what type
- The results of any tests carried out and what these mean
- Whether the form of arthritis that you have only affects your joints or whether other areas of your body might be affected. If so, which areas, how might they be affected and what signs should you look for?
- What course is your disease likely to take and what is the long-term prognosis
- What your treatment options are and how they work
- The risks involved in not being treated
- How soon you can expect to see any results from the various treatments prescribed
- Any possible side effects which might occur as the result of prescribed medications and what you should do about them
- What changes in your symptoms need to be reported to your doctor
- If changes in symptoms can be handled on your own, how should you manage them?
- How your condition will be monitored
- What happens if the proposed course of treatment does not work. Are there other options?
- Whether you need to make any changes to your lifestyle, and if so what type of changes
- Which exercises you should do, how often and for how long
- What you can do to protect your joints
- How you can learn more about your condition
- Whether there are any support groups that you can join
- Whether your children are at greater risk of suffering from the same condition either now or later on in life
- When you next need to see your doctor

If you have any other relevant concerns, such as in connection with fertility or pregnancy, or if you have relatives whose experience of the same condition either ended tragically or has led you to feel particularly fearful, then again, now is the time to raise them. You might also want to discuss alternative medicines or natural therapies which might help with your condition.

With any chronic condition, understanding is imperative, not only in terms of removing fear and stress, but also to allow you to achieve the very best quality of life. If there is anything at all that you are not clear about, be sure to raise it with your doctor.

Being Diagnosed with Arthritis

Because arthritis is such a common condition, it might be easy to think that being diagnosed with it would have little effect. As you will have seen from Chapter 3 of this book, however, even the most common forms of all have the potential to cause great suffering and to greatly affect the sufferer's quality of life. Some of the rarer but more serious forms can have even worse consequences and in a few cases they can even lead to fatality. Far from being a condition to be taken lightly, it is one whose diagnosis may cause you to feel shocked, fearful on many different levels, frustrated and even angry. These feelings, however, are all perfectly normal and natural and are certainly nothing to feel ashamed of.

Despite its ability to change lives and despite any initial feelings of helplessness, understanding the condition and the impact that it might have on your life and the lives of those around you is absolutely key to taking back control. Not just in terms of medical treatments and therapies, but also in terms of your lifestyle, your emotional and psychological well-being and your family, work and social life, there is in fact a great deal that you can do to preserve your quality of life and live as normally as possible. I will look at these issues in Parts II and III of this book.

No matter what the disease or condition, research has shown time and time again that those who confront chronic illness head-on and with a positive mental attitude fair much better than those who struggle with acceptance or who see their future as bleak. While your diagnosis may indeed have come as a shock, the attitude that you take forward with you into the future *will* dictate the extent of your suffering, and your attitude is something in which you do have a choice.

7

Aggravating Factors

As we have seen so far, the nature of the symptoms associated with the various forms of arthritis can vary quite considerably, as can their severity. What is fairly typical of many types of arthritis, however, is that sufferers experience periods when their symptoms feel either better or worse, and in some cases the disease can either go into complete remission quite spontaneously or it can be forced into remission through treatments and/or lifestyle changes.

The things which can aggravate arthritis are not just physical factors, but emotional ones too, and in this chapter I am going to look at some of those which doctors and sufferers themselves have found to be particularly influential in terms of determining the severity of symptoms.

Excess Weight and Obesity

Excess body weight and obesity are both causes and aggravating factors of a variety of different medical health problems, and they play a significant role in a number of forms of arthritis, notably the two most common, namely osteoarthritis and rheumatoid arthritis. As we have seen, they also contribute greatly to the development of other conditions which are sometimes associated with arthritis, such as diabetes.

Even in cases where excess weight was not a contributory factor to developing arthritis, weight gain can still become a problem once the disease starts to take hold. Not only can some of the medications used to treat the disease lead to weight problems, but so too can the curtailment of physical activities because of joint pain and stiffness.

When you bear in mind that every additional kilogramme of weight could put five times the stress on the joints, even a relatively small weight gain can have a significant negative impact on the joints, with the larger weight-bearing joints such as the hips and the knees being especially at risk. In osteoarthritis, this additional pressure can cause even greater mechanical wear of the cartilage and bone and lead to higher levels of pain, and in rheumatoid arthritis and other inflammatory forms of the disease, it can lead to increased swelling and soreness. For sufferers of psoriatic arthritis, not only does being overweight contribute to increased levels of joint pain, but it aggravates the associated skin condition too. In overweight women, for example, skin lesions in breast and abdominal folds are more common, but in either gender folds of skin are likely to lead to more rashes and greater discomfort and obese patients are likely to suffer a more severe form of psoriasis overall.

One of the very important things to remember about being overweight or obese is that the presence or increased risk of conditions such as high blood pressure or heart disease can seriously affect the range of treatments available to you, not just in relation to arthritis, but also for other illnesses and disorders. As you will see in Part III of this book, certain medications which can help to alleviate the symptoms of arthritis are contraindicated for those with other existing medical complaints, which could potentially limit your range of treatment options.

Diet and Food Allergies

Diet is a hugely important factor in arthritis, but not just because of the link with excess weight or obesity. Some sufferers find that certain foods and drinks seem to cause flare-ups in inflammation, although whether this is as a result of allergies to the particular items or whether these foodstuffs are genuinely pro-inflammatory in nature is not certain. What is the case, however, is that precisely which foods and drinks cause problems seems to vary from one individual to another. The following though, are some of the most often-quoted problem items:

- Red meat
- Pork
- Poultry
- Shellfish
- Fried foods
- Hydrogenated fats
- Eggs
- Dairy products – especially full-fat products
- Potatoes
- Tomatoes
- Peppers
- Aubergines
- Oranges
- Corn
- Wheat
- Oats
- Rye
- Processed foods
- Salt – other than sea salt
- White sugar
- Coffee
- Alcohol – especially beer
- Synthetic sweeteners
- Food additives, including colourings, flavour enhancers, stabilisers and preservatives

Although it can often be extremely useful to eliminate different elements from the diet entirely in the first instance and then reintroduce them to assess whether they are in fact causing a problem, it does not necessarily follow that sufferers have to avoid the offending foodstuffs completely thereafter. Some patients find that they are able to reintroduce these items into their diets quite successfully, albeit at lower levels. Do remember though, that if you do decide to try an elimination diet to help you identify problem foods, it may take two or three days after its reintroduction before it starts to aggravate your condition, so be sure to give it long enough to be able to determine the effects properly. Also, as arthritis symptoms typically come and go or vary in intensity, bear in mind that any variation in pain levels may be purely coincidental and so if you suspect a certain foodstuff of causing problems, it might be worth testing it more than once.

Alongside the things which sometimes cause painful flare-ups in arthritis sufferers, there are also certain foods and supplements which are believed to have an anti-inflammatory effect. Omega-3, which is naturally found at high levels in fish such as salmon, mackerel, tuna, herring and halibut, as well as in walnuts, walnut oil, flax seed and flax seed oil, can also be taken in supplement form and a dosage of at least two grams per day has been shown to have beneficial effects on the inflammation caused by arthritis. Cherries, blackberries, blueberries, raspberries and strawberries are also believed by some to have natural pain-relieving and anti-inflammatory properties.

It is always advisable to check with your consultant at your chosen pain management clinic, or the qualified nutritionist who forms part of your professional healthcare team before making changes to your diet. Those patients who suffer from diabetes or any other type of illness which has direct links with food and nutrition should be especially careful to follow the advice of their physicians.

Dehydration

As it is estimated that 60–70% of the human body is made up of water, taking in sufficient liquids is vital for overall health and well-being, regardless of whether you suffer from arthritis or not. Because, amongst other things, water helps to lubricate the joints, drinking eight tumbler-sized glasses of water every day can help to reduce the damage to cartilage in the case of osteoarthritis for example, and some also believe that it can guard against the painful inflammation of rheumatoid arthritis.

Drinking sufficient quantities of water is also important in terms of flushing out impurities from the body. In the case of gout, drinking plenty can help to prevent the build-up of uric acid and so prevent the uric acid crystals, which cause painful inflammation in the joints, from forming.

One question which is often asked in relation to the minimum intake of liquid into the body is whether that liquid has to be water. Although of course it does not generally hurt to drink the occasional glass of fruit juice or squash, because water does not contain sugars or additives such as colourings and flavourings, it is considered to be much more beneficial. Where tea and coffee are concerned though, it is advisable to drink these only in moderation, if at all. Recent studies have shown that those who drink four or more cups of tea per day are at greater risk of developing rheumatoid arthritis and, when tested on rats, green tea was seen to increase the severity of the condition. A study which was conducted in Finland, meanwhile, indicated that coffee induces the production of rheumatoid factor, which of course is found in most rheumatoid arthritis sufferers but only 1–2% of healthy people. In addition, many sufferers themselves have found that tea and coffee tend to aggravate their symptoms, so it may be worthwhile eliminating these from your diet for a period of time to check what effects it has.

Physical Activity

Physical activity and exercise are extremely important considerations for arthritis sufferers and many have learned to their cost that avoiding them tends to aggravate their symptoms. Although it was once thought that resting arthritis-affected joints was the key to avoiding further damage, as anyone with the condition knows, sitting, lying or maintaining any position for too long only serves to increase pain and stiffness. However, the wrong types of activities carried out at the wrong times, such as those which put excessive strain on joints which are inflamed, can be equally harmful.

As I discussed under the heading of Excess Weight and Obesity, physical activity and exercise are vital for overall health and to avoid excessive weight gain. Not only this, but the release of endorphins (commonly described as nature's pain killers) which occurs when we exercise, helps to reduce pain as well as making us feel more alert and improving our mental state. If the right effects are to be achieved though, it is vital that the right types of activities are prescribed, that the patient is shown how to carry out exercises properly and that recommendations in terms of how often and for how long the activities should be carried out are followed.

Many patients with arthritis and other chronic pain conditions become frustrated with exercise. Because they do not see immediate results, they fail to continue with the recommended activities. Giving up, however, only leads to increased pain and stiffness and the greater potential for long-term disability and a poorer overall quality of life. Not only can less frequent activities such as travelling and going on holiday be affected, but even normal day-to-day tasks and simple pleasures such as kicking a ball around with the children. Work and the ability to continue earning a living can also become highly problematic if the necessary steps are not taken to remain as active as possible.

Multidisciplinary treatment programmes will almost invariably include recommendations for exercise and physical activity. Under the care of a trained physiotherapist, patients are shown how to carry out exercises in a way which is safe and which will cause no further damage to the joints. Usually these are carried out under direct supervision in the first instance, and then patients are given recommendations for continuing with their exercises safely at home.

Medications

It is almost certainly true to say that there is not a single prescribed or over-the-counter medication which does not have the potential to have adverse effects on at least some proportion of the population. Of course, when patients start taking different drugs for different conditions, or a range of different medications to tackle the different symptoms brought about by the same condition, there is an even greater chance of a less than beneficial reaction. This is one of the reasons why a holistic approach to treatment is invariably the best option, because all aspects of the treatment programme are supervised by a consultant who can see the complete picture and is able to adjust the programme as necessary.

Although many of the drugs used to treat arthritis do not normally bring about any short-term aggravation of symptoms, there are two groups which do have the potential to cause longer-term deterioration in the overall conditions of sufferers. As I mentioned earlier when I was discussing the bone-thinning disease osteoporosis, corticosteroids can reduce the amount of calcium which is absorbed by the body, causing bones to become weaker and more likely to fracture. For this reason, doctors will normally only prescribe them over a relatively short period of time and then wean the patient off.

Another group of drugs which is causing increasing amounts of controversy, however, is that which includes the bisphosphonates such as Actonel and Fosamax. These drugs are actually prescribed for the very purpose of preventing the loss of bone mass which is seen in sufferers of osteoporosis, but more recent studies have shown that even though these medications are highly effective in the short term, when taken for a period of five years or more, they may in fact increase the risk of fractures. Although there is no suggestion that bisphosphonates be removed from the market, great care is needed in terms of assessing the risk of fracture before these drugs are prescribed and, if the risk is high, then it may be advisable to avoid their long-term use.

Environmental Factors

As well as being suspected of being the initial trigger for some forms of arthritis, environmental factors such as the toxins in the air, in the food that we eat and even in the fillings in our teeth are believed by some to aggravate the symptoms of the disease, and particularly the autoimmune forms such as rheumatoid arthritis. One source, for example, points to tests carried out on rodents using the toxic element mercury, which altered the immune response to a particular infectious agent and increased both the incidence of autoimmunity and the severity.

Mercury is just one of the heavy metals that we are exposed to at much higher levels today than in previous centuries. Not only is it used as a base for the preservatives in some vaccines, but this highly toxic element can also enter our bodies via decaying amalgam dental fillings and through eating mercury-laden fish. As many of the symptoms of mercury poisoning are seen in at least some of the patients who have rheumatoid arthritis, there are those who think that the introduction of the element into our bodies might at least be responsible for worsening autoimmune disorders, even if it does not cause them.

In rheumatoid arthritis patients, it is thought that reduced levels of glutathione, which is produced by the liver and plays an important role in neutralising toxic substances, could be responsible for a build-up of toxins and the aggravation of symptoms which affect a whole range of the body's systems. Further studies are required, however, to ascertain precisely what effects substances such as heavy metals, pesticides and so on have on the human body in general and how they might contribute to the development or worsening of arthritis in particular. In the meantime, of course, both sufferers and non-sufferers of the condition are probably best advised to avoid exposure to toxins wherever possible, such as by choosing organic produce over non-organic.

Toxins, though, are not the only environmental factors which might cause painful flare-ups in people with arthritis, and heat, humidity and barometric pressure are three factors which are commonly reported by sufferers to affect the condition. Some swear by their ability to predict weather conditions on the basis of their symptoms, such as by an increase in pain levels before it starts to rain, and others have gone so far as to relocate to a different area of their home country or even abroad because of the beneficial effects of different types of weather conditions.

Although there is no conclusive evidence to suggest that weather conditions can affect arthritis symptoms, and indeed some studies have shown conflicting results, there are, however, several factors which might explain why some people seem to benefit from living in warm, dry climates or from high barometric pressure:

- As it relates to the human body, barometric pressure is the force exerted on the body by tiny particles of air. One theory claims that when the barometric pressure drops and there is less force on the body, this allows the body's tissues to expand, which in the case of an arthritis sufferer means that tissue which is already inflamed swells even further, thereby causing more pain
- Cold, rainy weather tends to encourage people to stay indoors, which typically means that they do not take the regular exercise which would help to keep their symptoms in check

- The weather affects our moods and cold, wet weather often makes us feel down, which in turn causes our pain thresholds to drop
- Our bodies need adequate levels of vitamin D to protect us from autoimmune diseases and to promote the growth of strong, healthy bones (vitamin D promotes the absorption of calcium). Very few natural foodstuffs contain vitamin D and one of our main sources is sunlight. In warm, dry climates where people are outdoors for much of the time, their bodies can maintain higher levels of the vitamin

On the other hand, however, you do not have to be an arthritis sufferer to know that heat and humidity can also cause the joints to swell. For someone who does suffer from the condition, therefore, this increased swelling could lead to a worsening of inflammation, rather than an improvement. Also, if temperatures and humidity become uncomfortably high, those living in hot climates can often be persuaded to stay indoors with the air conditioning switched on, which of course means that they are robbed of the beneficial effects of the sun, as well as those which come from regular outdoor exercise.

In much the same way that different people record different effects from the inclusion or exclusion of certain types of foods from their diet, so too do weather conditions seem to affect arthritis sufferers differently, so that what works for one person does not necessarily work for another. If you do find that your symptoms ease each time you visit a certain location, however, it is worthwhile giving considerable thought to making a permanent move and to ensure that you visit the location often and at different times of the year before making any commitment to the decision.

Something else which is also worth thinking about is your state of mind when you visit the new location. As we will see in just a moment, stress can have some quite significant physiological effects on the body and if you are typically stressed at home but more relaxed in the new location, for example because you are on holiday, any improvement in your symptoms may be related to this factor rather than the different weather conditions. Also, bear in mind that if you were to move and leave friends and family behind, your stress levels in the new location may well begin to rise and this might undo the benefits derived from being in drier, warmer conditions.

Stress, Anxiety and Depression

When we experience stress, certain chemicals are released into the bloodstream and the body undergoes physical changes which prepare us to deal with the stressful event. In situations where we feel frightened, angry or even exhilarated, for example, our bodies sweat in order to cool us down, blood is diverted from the skin and the internal organs to the muscles in preparation for our 'fight or flight' response and our pupils dilate to let in more light and help us to see more clearly. All of these things are perfectly normal, natural and healthy responses which help to keep us safe and usually once the danger has passed the body settles back down to its normal state.

When stressful situations and circumstances are prolonged and unrelenting, however, the effects on the body become harmful rather than helpful. The chemicals which are released into the brain and the body can not only result in high blood pressure, heart disease, anxiety and depression, but they can also lead to flare-ups in pain and inflammation. In people who suffer from chronic pain conditions what frequently happens is that a vicious cycle develops. The individual starts off by experiencing pain which then leads to the diagnosis of a chronic pain condition, which in itself causes stress. As the person perhaps struggles to accept the condition and as he or she comes to deal with the daily impact of pain, limited mobility, fatigue, dependence on others, changes to their working and social lives, altered financial circumstances and low self-esteem, so stress levels rise further. As this happens, muscles begin to tense and increased pain and worsening symptoms result, which in turn leads back to more stress. In addition, if it is allowed to continue unabated, stress can quickly lead to anxiety and depression which I discussed in Chapter 4, and the sufferer's quality of life can soon spiral downwards.

Learning how to handle stress is important for all of us, regard-less of whether or not we suffer from arthritis or some other type of chronic pain condition. Because arthritis sufferers have so many additional problems, worries and concerns which are directly related to the disease, however, and because stress plays such a huge part in aggravating pain and other symptoms, it is absolutely vital to find ways to deal with it, and this is something which I will look at in more detail in Chapter 23 of this book.

Keeping a Health Journal

As we have seen throughout the course of this chapter, the factors which can aggravate the symptoms of arthritis are not only many and varied, but in many cases they affect different people in different ways. One type of food, for example, might have a negative effect on one sufferer but none whatsoever on another. One person might benefit from being in a warm, dry climate while another might experience more severe symptoms. What all of this means, of course, is that taking a broad brush approach to treating arthritis and making general recommendations is often inappropriate. Not only do medical practitioners need to tailor treatment programmes to meet individual needs and circumstances, but sufferers themselves need to understand precisely what causes improvement to their symptoms or aggravates them.

One of the simplest but most effective ways to establish what causes flare-ups in pain and other symptoms is by keeping a health journal which allows you to identify patterns and to establish any improvements which might occur as the result of changes to various aspects of your treatment or your lifestyle. You might, for example, record:

- What you eat
- How much water you drink
- What physical activities or exercises you take part in
- The weather conditions
- What medications you take
- Your moods, feelings and emotions
- Any practical concerns that you are battling with, such as financial worries, concerns about children or difficulties at work
- Any noticeable changes in your symptoms

Keeping a health journal is not only useful from a practical perspective, allowing you to report changes to your healthcare professional so that any necessary adjustments can be made to your treatment programme and to identify the things which cause flare-ups in symptoms, but it also serves as a highly effective way to release stress and anxiety and to give you an outlet for positive emotions and the opportunity to record your dreams, goals and aspirations for the future. Try to update your journal on a daily basis because leaving gaps for days or weeks on end will make it much more difficult to identify patterns. If your arthritis makes writing painful, then consider investing in a good ergonomically-designed pen to use for the purpose.

Of course, although writing a health journal can go a long way to providing an outlet for emotions in itself, it is important to read over what you have written on a regular basis with a view to spotting patterns. As these begin to emerge, try to think creatively about adjustments that you could make to your lifestyle to avoid negative consequences. Instead of seeing these things as being limitations and restrictions to your life, try to view them as opportunities to do things differently and approach them with a positive and determined attitude.

8

Top Arthritis Myths

Perhaps because there are so many different forms of arthritis, or perhaps because the severity of symptoms can vary enormously from one sufferer to the next, various myths have grown up around this condition. Although I hope that this book will help to dispel most if not all of these, here is a brief summary of some of the most common ones and the facts which actually underlie them.

Myth 1 – Arthritis is an old person's disease
Arthritis affects people of all ages, from babies and children to the more elderly members of the population. Although the most common form of arthritis, osteoarthritis, predominantly affects people over the age of 50, and the second most common, rheumatoid arthritis, tends to strike between the ages of 40 and 60, a number of other forms of the disease have a typical onset age which is much younger. In the UK, it is estimated that around 12,000 children under the age of 16 and around 27,000 below the age of 25 are affected by one of the different forms of the condition.

Myth 2 – If I just ignore my symptoms, they will clear up on their own
Literally millions of people around the world suspect that they might be suffering from a form of arthritis, but fail to seek medical attention in the mistaken belief that the symptoms will simply clear up on their own without any treatment or changes to their current lifestyles. Not only is this a myth, but it is actually quite a dangerous one which can lead to sufferers becoming permanently disabled and experiencing severe complications, which in some cases affect internal organs such as the heart, lungs and

kidneys and can even lead to premature death. Many forms of arthritis require early and aggressive treatment if their effects are to be controlled and so seeking expert medical advice is imperative.

Myth 3 – Arthritis only causes a few aches and pains

Although pain and inflammation of the joints are some of the main symptoms of arthritis, as I mentioned above, some forms of the disease have the potential to affect various other parts of the body and can lead to permanent damage to the primary organs, including kidney failure and blindness. Even in cases where only the joints are affected, patients can be left with permanent disability or at the very least suffer severe restrictions to their lifestyles if they do not seek appropriate treatment.

Myth 4 – My mother has arthritis, so I will get it too

Although there is some evidence that certain types of arthritis do appear more often in some families than in others, and even though certain genes are sometimes present in large proportions of the sufferers, there is no guarantee that just because a close family member has the condition that you will develop it too, or that you will pass it on to your children. The precise causes of arthritis are not fully understood at present and even though it may turn out to be the case that certain factors predispose certain individuals to particular types of arthritis, there may be a number of different factors which trigger the development of the disease in some and not others.

Myth 5 – As there is no cure for arthritis, there is no point in seeking medical help

While it is quite true that there is no cure for arthritis, there is much that can be done to help alleviate the symptoms of the condition, to improve the sufferer's overall quality of life, to slow down the progression of the disease and to avoid potentially dangerous complications from arising. As more and more is learned about arthritis, so new medications and therapies are being developed, and when these are combined to form a multidisciplinary treatment programme, much needless pain and suffering can be avoided. In some cases, arthritis can even be driven into complete remission through appropriate treatment strategies. At the very least, the disease can be controlled and managed so that it has a minimal impact on the life of the sufferer and those around him or her.

Myth 6 – The drugs used to treat arthritis cause too many side effects

All prescribed and over-the-counter medications have the potential to cause side effects in some people and this is no less true for arthritis medications than any others. Having said this, however, many people experience few or no ill-effects and a trained and qualified doctor who specialises in arthritis will monitor the drugs that you are taking to assess their effectiveness and to identify any side effects as a result of their use. If this is the case and the side effects outweigh the benefits of taking the medication, then the doctor will be able to try you on different drugs or make other adjustments to your treatment programme to help alleviate your arthritis symptoms. In most cases though, where side effects are experienced, these tend to be low level and are more than compensated for by the relief that they provide.

Myth 7 – Pregnancy makes arthritis symptoms worse

Actually, in many cases the reverse is true. In an estimated 70–80% of cases, the symptoms of arthritis subside during pregnancy and some women go into complete remission. Typically, however, the symptoms do return after the birth.

Myth 8 – Losing weight after being diagnosed with arthritis does not help

Excess weight or obesity can not only be an enormous factor in terms of the likelihood of developing arthritis, but it can also contribute greatly to the severity of symptoms and the rate of progression of the disease. Achieving an optimum weight for your height and build through diet and exercise is key to relieving unnecessary pressure on the joints, as well as to ensuring overall health, and it could even make the difference between ultimately having to face joint replacement surgery or not. In fact, because of the high cost of these operations, if you do not bring your weight down to within specified limits, you may not even qualify for surgery on the National Health Service in the UK. In addition, the increased risks which are associated with obesity may preclude the prescription of certain medications, thereby further limiting your treatment options.

Myth 9 – Exercise causes arthritis symptoms to worsen

Although it was once thought that using the affected joints would bring about further degeneration and lead to greater levels of pain, in fact exercise and physical activity are absolutely key to reducing pain levels and maintaining mobility. Although there are certain occasions when stepping down physical activity is advisable, such as where there is significant and active inflammation, in most cases arthritis symptoms respond extremely favourably to regular exercise. It is, however, important to take advice from a medical practitioner who is qualified and experienced in the treatment of arthritis so that you properly understand what type of exercise and physical activity is likely to be beneficial and so that you can learn how to carry out these activities safely.

Myth 10 – My GP is the best person to treat my arthritis

Arthritis is a complex condition which takes many different forms and which shares some of its symptoms with a whole variety of other illnesses. This often makes it very difficult for anyone who is not a specialist to diagnose the particular type of arthritis quickly, which can of course lead to delays in treatment and unnecessary further suffering.

When it comes to the treatment itself, unless your GP happens to be an expert in arthritis, the chances are that he or she is unlikely to be fully up-to-date with all the latest research and the new methods of treatment which are continually being developed, which again could mean that you do not have the opportunity to benefit from the most effective medications and therapies. Another extremely important consideration, however, is that in order for you to gain access to the wide variety of specialists that you might need, your GP will have to refer you elsewhere and no single person will be closely overseeing the various aspects of your treatment. In a practical sense, what this means is that one specialist might recommend a course of treatment which has a negative impact on another aspect of your treatment, but as there may be little or no communication between the two specialists, it will be almost impossible to gauge what has caused the negative impact or how the overall treatment plan can take this into account.

By dealing with a specialist in pain management who has the facilities to offer all of the necessary aspects of treatment under the same roof, however, it is possible to take the holistic approach to treatment which has proved consistently to be far more effective. In such an environment, not only do you have the benefit of a consultant to oversee your case, but trained and qualified specialists from a variety of fields which take into account the physical, emotional and psychological aspects of the disease.

Part II

Living with Arthritis

9

The Physical, Emotional and Psychological Impacts of Arthritis

Something which has probably become quite evident in the course of reading this book so far is that arthritis, in common with many other chronic pain conditions, is not just a disease which affects the physical body. In many cases, sufferers find that the condition impacts on their emotional and psychological well-being and has entirely unexpected consequences in terms of their family, social and working lives, their relationships, their image, their independence and their sense of self-esteem. In Part II of this book, therefore, I want to take a look at what it means to live with arthritis, because as they say, 'Forewarned is forearmed'. In this part and in Part III, you will also find numerous tips which I hope will go a long way to helping you to manage your condition and achieve the maximum quality of life possible.

Physical Restrictions

Although the symptoms of arthritis can sometimes be mild, even in these cases the condition can impose physical restrictions on the sufferer's lifestyle. Even the simplest of daily tasks which were once performed with ease can become difficult, painful and exhausting, making today's hectic lifestyles impossible to keep up with and extremely frustrating. Here are just a few of the everyday physical activities which many arthritis sufferers find problematic:

■ Walking even relatively short distances without experiencing pain or feeling extreme tiredness

- Maintaining a sitting, standing or lying position for any length of time, such as when attending the cinema, waiting in a queue or trying to sleep
- Climbing stairs
- Reaching high cupboards or shelves
- Opening jars
- Doing housework
- Driving, especially if the driving position is uncomfortable or where there is pain on turning the head
- Getting into and out of vehicles or being a passenger in a car even on relatively short journeys
- Using public transport, especially where bus stops or train stations still leave a long walk at either or both ends of the journey, where there is no guarantee of a seat and where there are high steps which need to be negotiated to embark and disembark
- Lifting and carrying, such as carrying shopping bags
- Decorating or doing DIY jobs around the house

The list, of course, could go on and on and until you actually find yourself faced with dealing with everyday life as an arthritis sufferer, it is hard to imagine just how many activities we all normally take for granted. Exercise can help greatly to overcome physical limitations and to restore mobility. But where certain restrictions still remain or where painful flare-ups in your condition make things feel temporarily unmanageable, there are a range of people, products and services which can help you to work around any restrictions that your condition might place on you. Here are a few practical tips to consider.

1. Try to visit shops, banks or anywhere else where you might have to stand in a queue during the quieter times of the day.
2. If you are doing anything which involves sitting for any length of time or carrying out a repetitive activity which uses the affected joint(s), set yourself an alarm to remind you to get up and move around or change activity every 15–20 minutes so that you do not become stiff and sore.
3. Re-arrange, or get someone else to re-arrange the contents of your cupboards so that the things that you need most are within easy reach.

4. If climbing stairs is difficult, then move the things that you need most downstairs or make a point of collecting up the things that you will require during the course of the day and bring them downstairs when you first get up.

5. De-clutter your home to make chores such as dusting and vacuuming quicker and easier, and if standing for long periods to do jobs such as ironing causes pain and discomfort then do them sitting down instead.

6. If you find that the early part of the day leaves you feeling most stiff and tired, then put off anything which requires too much effort until later.

7. Try to pace your activities and do a little bit often rather than storing everything up for the days when you feel slightly better and risking overdoing things.

8. Even the simplest chores may take longer to complete than they used to, so try to schedule your activities so that you allow yourself sufficient time without having to over-exert yourself or rush and potentially cause yourself an injury.

9. Prioritise your tasks so that even if you do not manage to get everything done, at least you will have attended to the most important things.

10. If you find it difficult to get in and out of the bath or shower or use the toilet, consider investing in a handrail to minimise the chances of accident and injury.

11. If arthritis affects your hands, then consider replacing any taps which require turning with lever taps.

12. Investigate automatic gadgets for opening tins and jars.

13. Even tasks such as carrying dinner plates to the dining room table can be difficult if you have problems with your hands, so consider buying a trolley for moving things around.

14. Only put as much water as you need into pans and kettles to keep down the weight and avoid accidents.

15. If you find bathing or washing-up difficult using hand-held sponges, then try using long-handled sponges or loofahs instead.

16. If you have a telephone with small buttons or a heavy receiver, consider swapping it for a light, hands-free set with large buttons or a touchscreen and then programme the numbers that you use

most into the phone memory to avoid having to dial long numbers each time you need to make a call.

17. If reaching the telephone before the caller hangs up is a problem, then set up an answerphone service so that you can call back or use a hands-free device that you can carry with you.

18. Make sure that you always have one telephone handset upstairs and another downstairs to avoid running up and down.

19. If you find it difficult to operate the locks in your home because of their height or because small keys are hard to turn, then consider changing them.

20. If grocery shopping is a painful and difficult ordeal, then consider ordering online and having it delivered.

Even though you have done things in a particular way for years on end, think creatively about how you can do them differently and more efficiently in the future. Also, do be aware that some social service authorities may be able to provide you with specialised equipment to help make your life easier and more manageable if you have severe physical restrictions, so find out what is available and how to go about arranging it.

Emotional Distress

Pain, far from being just a physical experience, is an emotional experience too. Living with a chronic pain condition, not to mention dealing with the shock of being diagnosed with such a condition and trying to come to terms with what might be a vastly changed lifestyle can play havoc with your feelings. Fear, frustration, guilt, anger and a whole host of other emotions can quickly and easily rise to the surface, which can not only lead to lashing out at those nearest and dearest to you, but also to blaming everything on your condition.

The first point worth making here is that an emotional response to discovering and living with a long-term medical condition is perfectly normal, natural and understandable. While there is no reason to beat yourself up for the feelings that you experience, however, it is important to understand that your ability to identify where these emotions are coming from and how to handle them will make an enormous difference in terms of acceptance and moving forwards with minimal disruption to your lifestyle. A 'poor me' attitude, whilst it might encourage the sympathy of others, will do nothing to make you feel empowered and in control of your own life. Again, here are a few tips to help you come to terms with and deal with your emotions.

1. Emotions are complex things and sometimes a current event or situation, such as discovering that you have arthritis, can dredge up all kinds of feelings from the past which are in no way related to the illness. Really stop to think about the emotions that you are experiencing and ask yourself honestly where they originated. If they lie in unresolved issues from the past, it might help to seek counselling or psychotherapy to help you to better understand and deal with them.

2. Although your emotions might seem quite overwhelming, always keep in mind that feelings cannot hurt you. Try not to be afraid of them, but instead face them head on and determine that they will not be allowed to control you.

3. Blaming everything on your condition and focussing all of your attention on it will not help you to get on with your life. Although it might be unreasonable to recommend that you think of having arthritis as an opportunity, at least try to think of it as nothing more than a situation over which you have a considerable degree of control.

4. Bottling up emotions can be extremely damaging and trying to do so can easily lead you into depression. While it is important not to engage in unrestrained expression of your feelings, it is vital that you find ways to express yourself appropriately. Writing things down can often be a great way to exorcise the demons within and to express things which might be better left unsaid, so try keeping a diary or including your feelings and emotions in your health journal. The very act of getting them down on paper can be immensely cathartic.

5. Alternatively, talk to someone, whether it be a trusted friend or family member, or a fellow sufferer or advisor from one of the arthritis associations. Even communicating with a fellow sufferer

through an online forum can provide immense relief and comfort, especially as you know that they understand what you are going through. Do, however, avoid making arthritis your sole topic of conversation, as not only will others soon become tired of the subject, but you are likely to fall into the temptation of wallowing in self-pity.

6. Negative emotions are extremely stressful, so try to find ways to relax. I will come back to the issue of controlling stress in Chapter 23 where you will find a range of helpful suggestions.

Psychological Damage

The prolonged stress of dealing with a chronic pain condition can have severe effects on our psychological health, not only changing how we view certain situations and events, but also how we respond to them. As I have said, sometimes the feelings associated with learning that you have arthritis might be a throw-back to feelings experienced in other traumatic circumstances in the past, while in other cases they might be directly related.

When feelings of hopelessness and despair start to get the better of us, not only does this impact on our physical well-being, but potentially on every aspect of our lives. Work, relationships and hobbies can all suffer greatly, and sometimes even irrecoverably, as our lives spiral out of control. In some cases, the anxiety and depression which follow can lead to harmful behaviours such as the abuse of illicit drugs or prescribed medications or alcohol abuse, all of which are designed to act as a crutch. Co-dependency is also common in families where one of the members suffers from a chronic pain condition. Clearly, however, these types of behaviours only add to existing problems rather than alleviating them and so seeking help for psychological difficulties is vital if negative trends are to be reversed.

Accepting help for psychological problems has, in the past, been seen as a sign of weakness, but increasingly people have come to understand the value of counselling and psychotherapy in terms of achieving greater self-awareness and acquiring the tools for long-term recovery. Men in particular still sometimes struggle with the idea of reaching out for professional help, but without this they condemn themselves to a life in which depression is likely to keep recurring.

As I mentioned earlier, although not in every case, sometimes a holistic approach to treating chronic pain conditions such as arthritis requires more than simply addressing physical symptoms. Where psychological issues do raise their heads, these need to be addressed as part of an all-encompassing treatment programme if the individual concerned is to be restored to a state of physical, emotional and psychological health.

One of the most effective types of therapy used in dealing with chronic pain conditions is known as cognitive behavioural therapy or CBT for short. CBT is a talk therapy which seeks to increase self-awareness and helps individuals become more conscious of the thoughts and feelings that they experience (cognitive), as well as dealing with what are often the self-defeating behaviours used to cope with them (behavioural) in order to set up healthier and more productive patterns.

10

Acceptance Issues

The five stages of grief was a theory which was first introduced in 1969 by Swiss-born psychiatrist Elisabeth Kübler-Ross in her book entitled *On Death and Dying*. In this book, she described a five-stage process by which people deal with grief, particularly when they are faced with being diagnosed with a terminal illness or the loss of someone close to them. The Kübler-Ross model, as it is more formally known, is not just useful in understanding how we deal with the process of grieving in these circumstances, however, but also in comprehending the feelings associated with the diagnosis of a chronic illness.

The five stages of grief which Dr Kübler-Ross outlined and which are still widely accepted by psychologists and psychiatrists today are ones that every human being must go through in order to heal and move forwards. The five stages are:

- Denial
- Anger
- Bargaining
- Depression, and
- Acceptance

The reason why I have deliberately not numbered the different stages is because not everyone moves through them in the same order and it is quite common to move backwards and forwards through the stages before finally completing the process. For some people, this might take a relatively short period of time, whereas for others it could take much longer, but however long it takes, all of the stages must be completed for healing to take place.

When faced with a diagnosis of arthritis, whether it be one of the more common forms of the disease, such as osteoarthritis or rheumatoid arthritis, or one of the rarer but potentially more serious types such as polymyositis, dermatomyositis or systemic scleroderma, denial can often be the first feeling to be experienced. While in some cases this stage is quickly passed and sufferers readily accept the illness and begin to focus on making the best of their situations, in others it can take longer or they can become stuck completely. Even despite being told by their doctors of the potential outcomes of the disease, these individuals do not truly accept that these things could happen to them and so they continue blithely on their way, sometimes even failing to take the prescribed medications, to carry out the recommended exercises or to make the necessary changes to their lifestyles which would help to minimise the risk of further damage to their joints and make their lives easier and more bearable.

The anger stage is often characterised by the words 'Why me?' Especially if the form of arthritis with which the sufferer has been diagnosed is a rare one or if the individual is younger than the average age range for the condition there can be a huge sense of injustice and this anger often helps to fuel any feelings of denial. While in some cases the anger may be directed outwards at the disease itself, at the people who are closest, at the world at large or even at God, in others the sufferer might blame him or herself for having the condition.

The third stage of grief identified by Elisabeth Kübler-Ross is bargaining, although some people replace this with fear. Both though, are perfectly relevant and can be seen as interlinked. Bargaining is when the sufferer begs or prays for the situation to be different, and during this stage it is not uncommon for people to try and make deals with God or their higher power to take the illness away. They might, for example, pray that if the situation is reversed, they will take better care of themselves in the future. Of course, what lies beneath the bargaining process is fear of the prospect of living with a condition which cannot be cured and of how it might change the sufferer's life in the future. Fear, however, typically comes from a lack of understanding and so learning about the disease is vital if the individual is to take back the control of his or her own life. It can also arise though, when someone doubts their own ability to deal with the illness. The world, however, is full of people who have not only lived through much worse, but triumphed in spite of, and sometimes because of their illnesses, so learning how to put the illness into perspective can often be key to moving through this stage.

Depression can often be an issue as people begin to realise that they are no longer able to do the things they used to do and as the extent of the limitations and restrictions on their lives become increasingly evident. Feelings of inadequacy can begin to arise and these in turn can lead to withdrawal and self-isolation. Concentrating on those activities or goals which remain unaffected by the illness can often help to overcome these feelings.

The final stage of the process, acceptance, is what allows us to move on successfully with our lives, but many people come unstuck at this point because they fear that accepting their illness means surrendering to it. In fact though, what it really means is saying, 'I don't like having arthritis, but I can live with it' and then controlling the disease through positive thinking and the willingness to take on board the recommendations and the changes which will help to restore a reasonable quality of life. It is about being ready to take up the challenge and even seeing a positive side to the situation. Many people with chronic illnesses, for example, take up new hobbies and interests or even new careers which they would not have considered had it not been for their conditions. Others develop whole new networks of friends as a direct result of their illnesses or find new, more efficient ways of doing things which, even without the disease, would have made their lives easier or more productive. For some, the mere reminder of their own mortality encourages them to take chances and do things they would only have dreamed of doing otherwise.

As human beings, most of us tend to grow up with an expectation that everything in life should be rosy and that we are somehow unfortunate if we happen to encounter difficulties along the way. In his highly-acclaimed book *The Road Less Travelled*, however, author and psychiatrist Dr M. Scott Peck begins with the truism 'Life is difficult'. No matter whether we are rich or poor, where we live in the world or whether or not we have arthritis, life is difficult for everyone, which is why we often hear the saying 'It's not what happens in life but how we deal with it that counts'.

Having arthritis does not define who you are as a person. It is an illness which may very well affect various aspects of your life but is still only part of your life as a whole. If you allow it to take control and to eclipse all the good, it will happily do so, but never forget that you do have a choice as to whether you let this happen. Everywhere there are wonderfully inspiring examples of human beings who have triumphed over adversity, such as those who have not only walked when doctors have told them that this would be an impossibility, but run marathons. These people are not exceptional beings, but 'ordinary' people like you and I. They have the same potential as everyone else, but instead of using the 1.5–2% of that potential which the average person uses, they reach deeper inside themselves to produce what look like miracles. There is nothing miraculous about them though and these things are within everyone's gift.

Being diagnosed with arthritis is life-changing, but how and to what extent it changes your life is a matter of choice. Accept it and move on with a positive attitude and you will fare better physically, emotionally and psychologically. Hold on to your feelings of anger and denial and your suffering will be greater.

If you find yourself stuck with negative feelings and unable to move past them towards acceptance, then it may be worthwhile seeking counselling or therapy. Far from being an admission of weakness, doing so is a demonstration of strength and the willingness to take control of your own life.

11

How Relationships Are Affected

Think back to the last time you had a heavy cold or a bout of the flu. You probably felt lousy and may even have taken a few days off work. You almost certainly did not feel up to carrying out your usual chores and even socialising with your friends was probably something that you preferred to avoid. The noise and the demands of your children for your attention might just have added to the misery and discomfort and you were probably a bit snappy with them and your partner. Even when you got better and returned to work, you almost certainly felt guilty about having taken time off and those suspicious looks from your boss probably did not help you to feel much better. And that was just a cold!

All illnesses have the potential to impact on our relationships with others. The more common ones which only last a few days typically have a mildly irritating effect but are still enough to cause arguments to break out or for people to be left feeling pushed aside. The more serious, terminal ones, on the other hand, often bring people closer together and encourage them to make the most of the time that they have left to enjoy one another's company and companionship. Chronic illnesses which are not normally life-threatening, however, in many ways have the potential to cause the most damage to relationships because there is no end in sight, only what seem like months and years of misery.

Our relationships though, are extremely important whatever our state of health. We humans are social beings who rely on the love, support and understanding of others and so preserving our connections with the people who play important roles in our lives is vital if we are not to be left feeling lonely and isolated. Where chronic illness becomes an issue in life, however, this is not always easy and so in this chapter I will look at the different ways that relationships can be affected by arthritis and what you can do to minimise those effects.

Relationships with Partners

Few if any relationships between same-sex partners or those of opposite genders are without difficulties, even at the best of times. When one of those partners has arthritis, however, this adds another dimension to the relationship and yet another area of potential conflict. Disagreements and misunderstandings can arise for all sorts of different reasons and around a variety of different concerns, including:

- Irritability caused by pain
- Frustration caused by limitations
- Expectations
- Feelings of helplessness
- Guilt
- Fear
- Preoccupation with the illness
- Poor communication
- Sharing of responsibilities
- Sex
- Loss of intimacy
- Loss of self-esteem and confidence
- Financial issues
- Social issues
- Expecting partners to be mind readers instead of asking for help

These, of course, are all problems which can arise from time to time in any close and intimate relationship, but where chronic illness comes into the picture, the issues are often magnified.

Another thing which can impact hugely on the relationships between couples where one is a sufferer of arthritis has to do with the difference between men and women's perceptions of pain. One study, for example, showed quite clearly that women make much better judgements than men in terms of the pain levels that their partners are experiencing. As the vast majority of people with arthritis are female, this suggests that a great many sufferers could be receiving, not only less empathy and understanding than they would like, but also less physical and emotional support. This disparity in terms of abilities to gauge another's pain can lead to misunderstandings and resentments, making effective communication and understanding between partners vital.

With so many different areas of potential conflict, but also the need for both parties to avoid treading on eggshells, here are some useful tips to aid effective communication and maintain harmonious relationships.

1. Being diagnosed with arthritis is not a minor thing and it is not uncommon for sufferers to become preoccupied with their illness and to talk of nothing else. Talking, however, can either take the form of whingeing and complaining about symptoms or it can address the underlying fears and concerns about the illness. Try to remember that there are other things in your life which are important other than having arthritis and also aim to discuss your real fears, even though these might be difficult to face. Other people cannot easily relate to your symptoms, but they can understand fears which revolve around how your future is likely to shape up or about the relationship itself.

2. Although partners can become quite good at intuiting one another's needs without any verbal communication needing to take place, remember that your needs have changed. If you need help or support from your partner, ask for it directly rather than waiting for it to be offered.

3. Even though pain, limited mobility and fatigue might be plaguing you, try to avoid snappiness and irritability with your partner as often this only leads to counter-attacks and full-scale arguments. Take a moment to think about what is really troubling you and then express it rationally.

4. Particularly if there are no visible symptoms of your condition, it can be hard for your partner to appreciate what you are going through. Without forcing it down his or her throat, try to ensure

that your partner has access to reliable and objective information about the disease so that there is less chance of them thinking that you are exaggerating your symptoms or simply trying to dodge unpleasant chores and responsibilities.

5. For yours and your partner's sake, always try to approach your condition with a positive attitude. People are usually much more inclined to help others when they can see that they are doing everything possible to help themselves.

6. When one partner is in what might be severe amounts of pain, maintaining a physical relationship can become difficult and so often requires a little more thought and creativity. Remember that if the evenings see you feeling overtired or wracked with pain, sex does not have to be restricted to this part of the day and if certain positions cause you discomfort then there are plenty of others which might not.

7. Some of the medications which might be used to treat arthritis or any associated medical conditions may have an impact on sexual libido. If this is the case, do not feel embarrassed to mention this to your doctor who may be able to prescribe an alternative drug.

8. Remember that sexual intimacy does not have to involve full intercourse. If you find that maintaining a normal sex life is impossible because of the pain, then try experimenting with oral or manual sex or simply enjoy giving one another a body massage.

9. If sexual difficulties do arise, do not just ignore them in the hope that they will go away of their own accord as this is only likely to cause bitterness and resentments to grow. Talk to your partner about any concerns or insecurities that you might have in order to maintain a close bond.

10. Sometimes when people are in constant pain and hobbling around like someone twice their age, it can reflect on their self-esteem and on how desirable they feel. Partners can help by showing that they still see the sufferer as a sexual being, by offering reassurance in the form of genuine compliments or even by buying an occasional treat to show their love and appreciation.

Relationships with Family

When young children in particular see a parent in pain and distress, not only can it make them feel frightened about what is going to happen to Mummy or Daddy, but guilty too. In their early years, children believe that the whole world revolves around them and so logic tells them that they are the cause of the illness. If the parent with arthritis is no longer able to take part in the kinds of activities which used to be shared with the child, this can also lead to feelings of rejection, which might manifest themselves in temper tantrums which are designed to seek attention or even to the child becoming quiet and withdrawn.

Another thing which can be an issue with younger and older children is that of taking advantage of the parent's illness. Although this is often not done at a conscious level, there can be the temptation for them to see the parent as weak in every sense and so to start pushing their luck or undermining the parent's authority.

Again, here are a few tips to bear in mind when dealing with arthritis and raising a family.

1. Try to keep things at home and with your children as near to normal as you can manage. Children derive much of their security from routine and many and frequent changes can be extremely unsettling for them.
2. Explain your condition to your children in simple terms that they can understand but which will not worry or frighten them. With younger children in particular, offer reassurance that they are in no way to blame for your arthritis.
3. Chronic illness can often cause us to reassess our priorities in life and children can take on even more importance than they did previously. Try not to let these feelings cause you to become too lax in terms of discipline as this will only store up problems for the future and will do nothing to benefit the child.
4. If some of the activities that you used to share with your children are no longer possible, find alternatives that you can manage. Children are normally far more concerned with having your attention and you being there for them than with the precise nature of the activities that you share.

5. Pace yourself and prioritise your activities so that you can spend quality time with your children. If that means leaving some of the housework until another time, then let it wait.

6. With older children, give them a few simple chores to do around the home. Not only will this help you by cutting down your workload, but it is a valuable exercise to teach them responsibility and to help them appreciate that you need their support.

7. Try not to let pain or the frustration caused by limited mobility lead you to snap at your children. Unlike adults who can usually work out for themselves what is at the root of your irritability, children can often take their parents' moods personally and blame themselves even though they are not at fault.

8. Do not forget that your children may be concerned about their own chances of suffering from arthritis in the near or more distant future. Make sure that you understand whether the particular type of arthritis that you have been diagnosed with is one which commonly runs in families, as well as the implications of genetic factors. If it helps, take your child along to one of your doctor's appointments and ask him or her to help you explain.

9. Beware of talking about aspects of your illness that you have not mentioned to your children with friends or family members whilst the children are within earshot. It is amazing what children sometimes manage to overhear and if things are taken out of context and misunderstood or if the child feels that he or she has been lied to, it can create enormous problems later on.

10. Remember that if you are going to be fit and well enough to look after your family, you need to look after yourself too. Be sure to get enough rest.

Of course, children are not the only family members who are likely to be touched by your illness. Your own parents, grandparents, brothers, sisters, aunts, uncles and cousins are all people that you might want to turn to for understanding and support and who are likely to be concerned about you. One of the most difficult things with family members, however, is the fact that they can often be full of 'good' advice which they are keen to share. In some cases that advice might not come from personal experience or a reliable source, but nevertheless they can still take quick offence if you choose not to take it. In addition, if family become overly concerned, there can be a sudden need to take care of you which you might find overwhelming or see as interference.

1. Explain your condition simply and unemotionally and point your relatives in the direction of further information if they want to learn more.
2. Tell them what your treatment involves and the things that you are doing to help yourself and if you need their help, ask for it directly.
3. If you neither need nor want help from your relatives but it is offered anyway, thank them for the offer, decline politely and offer your reassurance that everything is under control, but do not feel obliged to accept. At the same time, however, try to bear in mind that they may actively want to assist you, rather than feeling helpless.
4. Although your relatives may be close to you, try not to use them as a means of venting your negative feelings and remember that they have lives too.

Relationships with Friends

For many people, their friends are even more important than their family members, but even the close bonds of friendship can be put under strain when one gets sick. Where once you may have been able to go places together or even pop round to one another's houses regularly for a cup of coffee and a chat, these things might become more difficult if they require walking, using public transport or driving. As you turn down invitation after invitation and your friends begin to feel pushed out, contact and communication can become less and less frequent until eventually the friendship dissolves.

1. As with your partner and family members, explain your condition and your treatment simply and unemotionally to your friends and let them know how it affects your daily life. Again, if they want further information, then point them in the right direction.

2. Friendships are truly precious, especially because they are not born of blood ties and obligation but of choice. Even though it might sometimes feel like a monumental effort to get together, try to make it anyway, otherwise not going can become a habit and you could soon find yourself becoming very isolated. If you really are not up to it, be sure to remind your friend to ask again next time.

3. Getting together with friends can be a wonderful escape from the demands and concerns that we face at home, so try not to take all of your problems related to arthritis along with you. Remember, your friends need to know that you are interested in them too.

4. When we see the people that we care about in difficulties or in pain, one of the very worst feelings is that of helplessness. Your friends may have their own families and lives to think about, but if they want to help you out occasionally, then let them.

5. Particularly if your friends are of a similar age to you, bear in mind that your experience might raise fears in them about their own health and even cause them to keep their distance. Try not to complain or exaggerate your symptoms or problems when you are in their company.

6. Chronic illness can sometimes be a test of who your real friends are. You may find that some of those from your circle drop out on hearing about your arthritis and this can happen for a number of reasons. Think carefully about whether you want someone in your life who ducks out at the first sign of trouble and whether in the past this particular individual has put as much into the relationship as you have.

Advice for Carers

Often the people who care for arthritis sufferers are partners or close family members. Because these people have close personal ties to the individual, it can often make it extremely hard to express the frustration, resentment and anger which sometimes come with their responsibilities. Frequently eaten up with guilt for having these feelings at all, it is not uncommon for them to bottle up their emotions but then go on to experience emotional or psychological problems later on, and of course none of this does anything to help their relationship with the sufferer.

Some of the most common reasons why unpaid carers come to feel frustrated and resentful arise from:

- The feeling that they have no choice but to act as the primary carer
- Having to give up a job or career to take care of a loved one
- The stress of trying to juggle work and care-giving
- Having to cut back on hobbies and interests or socialising to fulfil the role of care-giver
- Feelings of isolation because so much time is spent in the company of the sufferer
- Feeling taken for granted or unappreciated
- Feeling guilty about neglecting other responsibilities such as to children or other family members

While it is important to recognise that these are all perfectly normal and valid reasons for negative feelings, there are a few things which many carers find it useful to remember.

1. Try to remember that as hard as it might be for you to care for your loved one, he or she is in an even harder place. Alongside the pain, discomfort and even deformity of the condition, the arthritis sufferer has to try and deal with the loss of independence and self-esteem and in some ways is reduced to a childlike state where they have to ask for anything they need. Having someone to help you dress or bathe might sound like being pampered, but in fact it is an extremely demeaning experience which makes people feel helpless and strips them of their dignity.

2. For both your sakes, use whatever resources are at your disposal to learn more about how the sufferer might be feeling so that you can better understand his or her frustrations, fears, worries and concerns. Sometimes these can be hard to accept from the sufferer directly, so seek out books, leaflets or factsheets or research some of the online forums where sufferers talk about their feelings.

3. Do not try to deny your negative feelings but be honest about them. These kinds of emotions are perfectly normal and natural and they do not make you a bad person.

4. Reach out to other carers through online forums or telephone helplines for advice and to share your feelings.

5. Do not be afraid to seek counselling if you are struggling with caring for a loved one. Often it is easier to talk openly and honestly to someone who is not directly involved in the situation and a counsellor will be able to work with you to find practical solutions to improve your situation.

6. Take a break from your responsibilities every now and again and let someone else take the strain. If you are caring for a family member, ask another relative or friend to fill the breach so that you can get away for a rest. If you are acting as care-giver to your partner, then take the opportunity to get away together to spend some quality time in each other's company or if you need a complete break, again ask someone else to step in on your behalf but do not feel guilty. Remember, you need to take care of your own health and well-being if you are going to be able to continue to care for your loved one.

12

Work Issues

As I mentioned in Chapter 2, Arthritis Care, the leading UK charity to support sufferers of the disease, states that 93% of people with arthritis have difficulty walking, 72% meet the legal definition of disabled according to the Disability Discrimination Act 1995 and 81% are in constant pain or are limited in terms of their ability to perform everyday tasks. Arthritis Research UK, meanwhile, estimates that up to 40% of people with rheumatoid arthritis lose their jobs within five years of the onset of the disease (in 75% of cases, job loss was directly related to their arthritis) and 14% give up work within one year of diagnosis.

Clearly, statistics such as these do little to reassure working sufferers of their ability to remain in employment should they wish to do so. Since these figures were produced, however, research carried out into the effects of advanced rheumatoid arthritis on employability in the USA seems to suggest that the situation may have improved considerably in more recent years, and undoubtedly this is at least in part due to developments in treatment and the greater understanding of the disease.

Inevitably there will be cases where arthritis has such a major impact that continuing in employment will prove impossible, but for most sufferers there are probably more options now than ever before for staying in paid work, and of course the rights of workers with disabilities are protected by law. In this chapter, therefore, I will look at some of the workplace considerations which are relevant to arthritis sufferers and some of the choices which are open to them.

Your Rights as a Worker

The Equality Act 2010, which replaced major parts of the Disability Discrimination Act 1995 in the UK (except in Northern Ireland), essentially protects workers from discrimination on the grounds of disability, but from 1 October 2010 it made it easier for individuals to demonstrate that they are disabled. One notable change, for example, is that people with disabilities no longer have to show that their condition affects a particular function, such as mobility, in order to qualify for protection from discrimination. In addition, however, the new law also protects individuals from 'indirect discrimination' which might put disabled people at a disadvantage in cases where policies or practices are applied equally and in the same way to everyone, as well as placing limitations on the types of questions which employers are permitted to ask in relation to health as part of the selection process.

Not just in the UK but in America too, employers are expected to make reasonable provisions and adjustments for their workers, even in cases where they are not formally registered as disabled. A worker who is extremely tall and could not work safely and comfortably using a regular-sized desk or chair, for example, would be expected to be provided with office furniture which was appropriate to his or her needs. These rights are, of course, protected under law for people with disabilities, with the only proviso being that any adjustments which are required should not impose undue hardship on the company.

What all of this means, therefore, is that irrespective of whether your arthritis developed during your time with your current employer and you wish to remain in your current job, or whether you choose to seek employment elsewhere at some point after being diagnosed with the disease, you have a right to expect that reasonable adjustments to the working environment are made which would allow you to carry out your duties safely and comfortably. These might include, for example:

- ■ Providing new work furniture or adapting existing furniture
- ■ Providing new equipment such as copy holders, telephone headsets, arm supports or wrist rests

- Adapting tools or equipment for your use
- Providing any necessary training which would enable you to use specialised or adapted equipment
- Rearranging furniture to make your workplace more accessible or relocating you to a more suitable work space
- Redistributing some of your work duties or tasks to other employees

Of course, the key here, as I have mentioned, is that any adjustments must be 'reasonable', so expecting an employer to install a lift or completely redesign a factory to meet your needs would clearly not qualify. Where reasonable adjustments would help you to continue in your work though, talk to your employer about the available options to see what can be done. Your employer may wish to bring in an occupational therapist to assess your needs properly and make suitable recommendations. Residents of the UK might also like to check out the website at www.direct.gov.uk for more information, or www.nidirect.co.uk in Northern Ireland.

Business as Usual

Although for some people with severe arthritis continuing in the same job may not be possible or even desirable, many others will want to continue working for their current employer. If this is the case, then alongside discussing any reasonable adjustments to your working environment, you might also wish to consider revised working arrangements which will help you to manage your condition and better accommodate your needs. One thing which many sufferers find extremely helpful, for example, is arranging to work flexible hours.

Nine to five working may still be the norm today, but increasing numbers of employers are quite happy to agree to flexible working hours, especially in what is a far more global marketplace. If you find that the earlier part of the day is when you experience most pain and discomfort then consider approaching your employer with a view to negotiating a later start and finish time. In some cases, employers might even be agreeable to you starting late on an 'as required' basis, but of course this will depend greatly on the nature of your role and responsibilities.

Another thing which many companies are much more open to

than ever before is work from home arrangements. With the high costs of maintaining premises and with so many of today's jobs involving the use of computers, many employers have actively encouraged their staff to work from home and this is a trend which is likely to become increasingly popular. Again, if you think that such an arrangement might better suit you, and particularly if you have a long and uncomfortable commute, then take it up with your manager to find out whether it would be possible. Even if you do not work from home every day, doing so on a couple of days per week can often help. If you are going to consider home working, however, do bear in mind that you will lose the social aspect of the workplace and that isolation can sometimes be an issue.

For some sufferers of arthritis, such as many of those with rheumatoid arthritis, the early stages can be when the disease is at its most aggressive, which may mean taking a period of sick leave. If you find that this becomes necessary, consider talking to your employer about a phased return to work when you are ready to go back so as not to present yourself with too great a challenge.

Another important thing to remember in all cases is that if you do need to take time off work because of your condition, whether it be just a day or two, a few weeks or even a period of months, it is vital that you meet your company's requirements in terms of calling in sick, providing doctor's notes and so on. You may be sick, but your employer still has a business to run, so be sure to keep him or her in the loop in terms of how long you expect to be off work so that alternative arrangements can be made in your absence and so that your own position is protected. In addition, always give as much notice as possible when you arrange healthcare appointments.

Different organisations of course have different policies in relation to special or disability leave, so be sure to check out where your employer stands on these issues. You may, for example, be able to apply for special leave for those times when you need to undergo treatment or you may be entitled to paid disability leave as well as sick leave. Never assume what your entitlements are, but check them out carefully so that you do not inadvertently leave yourself in a vulnerable position with your employer.

Changing Jobs

Depending upon the nature of your work or whether your employer is able to make reasonable adjustments to your working environment to accommodate the needs which arise as a result of having arthritis, you may find it impossible to continue in your existing job and need to seek alternative employment. As I mentioned earlier on in this chapter, if this is something you want to consider, then bear in mind that any new employer would also be expected to make reasonable provision for you to be able to fulfil your role and that you are protected from discrimination in the selection process.

Also, remember that there are strict limitations in terms of the questions that a prospective employer can ask you during the hiring or interview processes and that anything they do ask should be focussed on establishing whether you have the required skills and abilities to perform the role. Although recruiters are entitled to ask whether there is anything which would stop you from being able to perform the role given reasonable accommodation if required, they cannot ask outright whether you have any physical or mental disabilities, and nor are they entitled to approach your doctor with a view to acquiring your medical records without your express consent.

When considering a change of job, bear in mind that you do not have to go back into a traditional work environment and that there are several other options available to you. You might, for example, wish to take the opportunity to set up a business of your own that you can run from home, or take on freelance work which allows you to work as few or as many hours as you need to work. Websites such as www.elance.com and www.peopleperhour.com advertise thousands of jobs in a whole range of different fields which can be carried out on an internet-connected computer. Again, however, do think carefully about whether working from home is really for you as the lifestyle can be a lonely one, and also be realistic about the start-up costs of a business as the last thing you are likely to need is financial worries on top of your arthritis.

Giving Up the Daily Grind

Should your financial situation allow, you may wish to consider giving up work altogether, especially if you are already nearing retirement age. For some people this can bring immense relief and make living with arthritis very much easier, but careful consideration is needed. Especially if you have spent many years in the workplace, sometimes it can be hard to adjust to a life of leisure and there is the potential for levels of self-esteem to plummet if you take early retirement. In fact, even some people who are perfectly healthy experience the same feelings when they stop work at the normal retirement age and it is not uncommon for retirees to experience stress and isolation rather than the sense of freedom and enjoyment that they had anticipated.

13

Mobility and Disability Issues

Benefits and Allowances

Because the laws pertaining to benefits and allowances vary from country to country and are the subject of frequent changes, and because every individual's circumstances are likely to be entirely different, this is not an area that I intend to address in any detail in this book. Having said this, however, do bear in mind that you may be able to claim a range of different benefits to help with the extra costs of having arthritis. You may, for example, be entitled to disability or mobility allowances, attendance allowances to help with the costs of personal care, housing and tax benefits or benefits which are intended to supplement your income. In some cases, these might be means-tested, whilst in others they might be available to anyone who qualifies irrespective of earnings or employment status, so never assume that you are not entitled, but check it out on the internet or speak to your local authorities.

Something which is worth bearing in mind with claims for certain disability allowances is that you may have to undergo a medical assessment which involves an interview and sometimes a medical examination. The purpose of the assessment is not to diagnose or treat your arthritis, but to establish the extent to which your condition affects you. The results of the assessment are used to determine whether you are entitled to the allowance, which components of the allowance you may or may not be entitled to and how much benefit you will actually receive. In some cases, medical examinations are carried out even after you have started claiming the allowance with the aim of ensuring that you are receiving the right amount. Medical examinations are usually carried out in your own home or at a medical examination centre close to your home.

If you are in receipt of certain benefits, also do not forget that you may be entitled to certain other benefits such as disabled persons' travel cards or special parking permits or badges which allow you to park in normally restricted areas or which allow you to park free of charge.

Mobility Aids

For many people with arthritis, getting around without the use of a mobility aid is perfectly possible and might only involve some slight discomfort. For others, however, it can represent a significant challenge. Although accepting that you need some additional help might not be easy, if your quality of life is so impaired by your lack of mobility then it may be worthwhile discussing some form of specialised equipment with your physiotherapist.

One of the simplest and cheapest forms of mobility aids, of course, is a wooden or metal walking stick, and these can be ideal for providing extra stability. As well as the traditional sticks, there are also three-pronged models and quad canes, many of which are made from lightweight materials, and there are even canes which can be folded up and which are easy to carry around when not in use. For even greater stability, a walking frame is another option, although some people do find the models without wheels quite difficult to manoeuvre. Elbow or underarm crutches can be a useful option if putting some or all of your weight on your legs is a problem.

Quite understandably, most people would rather avoid the use of a wheelchair unless it became absolutely essential, particularly because long-term use can lead to muscle wastage and even greater weakness and instability. Even if this is the case though, do remember that there are certain times when a wheelchair can save enormous amounts of pain and discomfort, such as if you are going on holiday and find it difficult to get around the airport or if you are attending an exhibition which involves hours of traipsing around. Should you need to use one more regularly, however, then consider which areas of your body are affected so that you can choose the most appropriate model. A self-propelled model, for instance, might better suit someone who still has effective use of their arms and hands and of course these models can typically be folded up for easy transportation and are much lighter in weight. Electric wheelchairs, on the other hand, are typically better for those whose hands are affected but do bear in mind that if you travel regularly by car, then you will need a special ramp or lift to get the chair in and out, as well as a vehicle with sufficient headroom.

Where a wheelchair needs to be used indoors, you may need to consider special adaptations to your home. Doorways may need to be widened and work surfaces and light switches lowered, and you may even need to think about installing a stair lift. Particularly if you choose an electric wheelchair, which are usually extremely heavy, you may also need to think about changing your carpets or floor surfaces for something which can be glued down, as the movement of the chair across carpet can cause it to become quite badly rucked and rippled, which not only causes excessive wear but also represents a safety hazard for others in the house.

For those who work close to home or prefer to get out and about as often as possible and retain as much of their independence as they can, a powered scooter might be another alternative. Of course these, like electric wheelchairs, are more expensive to buy, but if you are entitled to certain disability allowances then you may be able to get some financial help towards the cost should you require it.

14

Image Issues

When we think about the deformities which are typically caused by arthritis, usually it is the little old woman with the gnarled fingers who comes to mind. Various forms of the disease, however, can cause deformity in a whole range of different joints and in some cases these can be quite severe. As we saw with systemic lupus erythematosus, sometimes the visible signs of arthritis are not even just confined to the joints, but can involve markings on the face or rashes and lesions on various parts of the body. In addition of course, arthritis might not just affect the way that you look, but also the way that you move, making your gait appear ungainly or clumsy.

Although it might be easy to imagine that younger sufferers of arthritis are the only ones to feel the effects of changes to their physical appearance, of course this is far from being the case. Men and women of all ages are normally very conscious of how they look and, especially if any changes are significant enough to cause other people to stare, this can be extremely upsetting and have enormous effects on the individual's self-esteem and self-confidence.

Probably the two most significant areas to be affected by changes in appearance caused by arthritis are clothes and relationships. Where the first is concerned, women in particular can find it especially distressing if they find that they can no longer wear pretty, feminine clothes which reveal their shapes. Often they resort to long or baggy clothing which hides misshapen joints or surgical scars but is not necessarily very flattering. Because anything with fiddly buttons, laces or zips can be difficult to manage, trying to find outfits which are easy to put on and take off, comfortable to wear and yet still look good can be extremely frustrating. Footwear too can be a problem, with heeled shoes or strappy sandals having to be replaced by flat, wide, 'sensible' footwear.

Thankfully, the range of clothing available today is much wider than in years gone by, not just in terms of style, but also in terms of size and shape. In addition, nowadays we have the benefit of being able to buy online from suppliers all over the world, rather than being restricted to our local High Street stores. Wherever you choose to shop for clothing, however, do remember that there are certain simple adjustments which can be made to make wearing them easier and more comfortable. Replacing small buttons with larger ones which are easier to handle or using Velcro fastenings, for example, are just two ways to make commercially available clothing wearable while still retaining a sense of fashion and style. Instead of viewing such adjustments as something necessitated by your condition, try to see it as an opportunity to express your creativity and to create a totally individualistic look.

For both youngsters and older singles, the area of new relationships is another one where image issues can cause great concern. On top of the worry that their condition might put prospective partners off because of any limitations that it might impose, there are also added anxieties connected with looking different. Often though, these fears are precisely what stand in the way of meeting someone new, because they lead to sufferers isolating themselves or becoming quiet and withdrawn when in company. Try not to let your condition stop you from getting out and about to spend time with your friends and meet new people, and also try to think positively and just be yourself. No matter whether a person has arthritis or not, confidence is always an attractive quality which draws other people, so try to resist the temptation to hide yourself away and become the proverbial wallflower.

Another thing to bear in mind is that people fear what they do not understand. When you do meet new people who you would be interested in having as a friend or partner, try to be open with them about your condition, both so that they do not feel afraid to put their foot in it when they talk to you, and so that they can understand how you might be feeling.

As I discussed in Chapter 11, sexual relations between existing couples can become a concern where one of the partners suffers from arthritis and this is no less the case for new couples. Take a look at some of the tips offered in Chapter 11 or speak to your healthcare provider if you feel able, but do remember that communicating with your partner is essential if you are to overcome confidence issues in this area. Another thing to remember is that practising safe sex, while important to anyone who is sexually active, is especially vital for those taking certain arthritis medications as some can cause harm to a developing foetus.

Probably one of the most important things to bear in mind with respect to image issues is that you are far from being alone. Most people, irrespective of whether they suffer from arthritis, are not entirely happy with the way that they look, but often what helps is to concentrate on highlighting your best features. Also, keep reminding yourself that anyone who is worth having as a friend or a partner will willingly see past any physical flaws to the person beneath, so let yourself shine as the unique individual that you are.

Parenting a Child with Arthritis

Particularly because arthritis is commonly thought of as an old person's disease, when a child is diagnosed with the condition it can come as a great shock to everyone concerned. Parents often report feeling angry, disbelieving and fearful at being presented with the news, and guilt, frustration and helplessness are extremely common. For those who have lived with a child who has been in pain and discomfort or suffered disturbing symptoms for some time without a proper diagnosis, however, it might even come as a relief for the disease to finally be given a name.

As the parent of a child with arthritis, one of the most important things to come to terms with is that you are not to blame for the illness and this is vital for two reasons. First of all, it will save you a great deal of unnecessary mental and emotional anguish, but secondly it will make it much easier for you to retain a sense of normality in respect to your family life. A parent who feels eaten up with guilt is much more likely to give in to a child who is sick and to make decisions which are ultimately not in the child's best interest in order to alleviate their own feelings.

Of course, no parent likes to see their child in pain and suffering and having a child with arthritis will almost certainly put more physical and emotional demands on the whole family. Understanding the disease, what to expect and how to manage it though, goes a very long way to making the situation more bearable and to ensure a better quality of life for the sufferer, the parents and any siblings. As well as speaking to your child's healthcare practitioner and reading the advice in this book, never feel afraid to reach out to the professional organisations which specialise in arthritis via their helplines or to other families and sufferers via online discussion forums or local support group meetings. Not only will these resources be able to provide you with valuable information and tips about how to cope with a child with arthritis, but developing a network of people who are in the same position as you can help greatly to undermine any feelings of isolation that you might experience.

Family Life

Trying to devote the same amount of time and attention to a number of siblings who each have different personalities and different needs could never be considered to be easy. However, when one of those children suffers from a long-term medical condition trying to get the balance right is even more challenging. The fact is though, that all things being equal, all of the children in the household, including the one who suffers from arthritis, is likely to grow up to have a life which involves going out to work, having a family and a social life, and so it is important that all are brought up in such a way that their physical, emotional and psychological needs are met and that they are prepared for the life ahead of them.

Keeping things as normal as possible is absolutely key to bringing up a child with arthritis and to ensuring that siblings do not feel in any way pushed out or neglected. Even the mandatory trips to the doctor can mean that the sick child spends more time with one or both parents and if the child's condition requires a hospital stay or that holidays or special events have to be cancelled, then this can quickly cause bitterness, resentment and jealousy to build up in brothers and sisters. While some of these things may be unavoidable, restoring the balance and including all of the family in as many activities as possible is vital if problems are to be avoided.

When a child with arthritis is feeling even slightly off par, it can often be tempting to curtail family activities such as trips to the park, days out or even just playing games at home. In some cases, sick children will even use their illness to avoid doing things that they simply do not want to do. As a parent, it is important to understand precisely what the child is capable of and when it is safe to go ahead, both for his or her own sake and the sake of the other children. Remember, children with arthritis need to learn how to grow up and live successfully with their condition and so allowing them to duck out of activities which they could take part in does not ultimately help, and of course it robs the other children in the family of a healthy social development too.

Maintaining a healthy lifestyle in terms of diet and exercise is important to any growing youngster, but for those with arthritis it can make a huge difference to the extent of any disability that he or she might suffer, as well as to the levels of pain and other symptoms. Although parents sometimes feel reluctant to enforce lifestyle changes on their children, actually most are very adaptable and, if the whole family is involved and allowed to have a say in making healthier choices, then often it is not as difficult as predicted. An activity such as swimming, for example, is typically excellent for someone with arthritis, but is equally as enjoyable for the other children too, making it ideal as a regular pursuit in which the whole family can enjoy some quality time together. Healthy food too, does not have to be boring, so have fun choosing healthier options that everyone will enjoy.

Social Life

Pain, tiredness and image issues are all things which can affect the social lives of children and teenagers with arthritis, but here again balance is key if they are neither to become isolated nor try to do so much that their symptoms are aggravated. Peer pressure, especially as they get older, and the feeling of missing out can sometimes make them feel obliged to join in with activities when they really do not feel up to it, so try to encourage them to listen to their bodies and to talk to their friends about adapting arrangements so that everyone can join in. Even something like suggesting a cinema or other meeting place which is closer to home, or some-where where your youngster is able to sit rather than stand could make the difference between whether they are able to go or not, and most true friends will be happy to accommodate.

For parents, one of the biggest difficulties can come from feeling over-protective, but just like non-sufferers, youngsters with arthritis need to develop social skills, to become independent and to have fun and relax. Encourage them to go out if they feel up to it, but also discuss with them the value of not overdoing things and having to pay the price later.

School Life

Although there may inevitably be times when the symptoms of your child's arthritis may prevent them from going to school, try to ensure that normal attendance is kept up if at all possible. As I mentioned earlier, children can sometimes use the symptoms of their illness to avoid doing the things that they do not want to do, and going to school can come pretty high on that list. Even if this is not the case, however, your child may very well need some extra consideration in terms of school life and there are a number of things that you might need to discuss with your child's teacher.

Medication is one issue that you will certainly need to mention to your child's school, because many have very strict rules in place which of course are intended to keep all of the children safe. If your child is younger or the school policy states that a member of staff must administer the medication, then be sure to write down the dosages and the times at which they are to be taken to avoid any confusion. Also, make sure that everyone understands whether the child needs to report to a particular staff member to collect the medication or whether the responsibility to deliver it lies with the school.

If your child needs to be absent from school for doctor's appointments, or if flare-ups in their condition make it impossible for them to attend, be sure to notify the school as appropriate.

Another key consideration which is often more relevant to secondary school students who need to move from classroom to classroom is timeliness. If your child has mobility problems which make it impossible to negotiate corridors and stairs in-between classes and still make it on time, or if doing so through the crush of other students makes it difficult, then ask whether he or she might be allowed to leave class slightly early. If there is a lift in the school which is normally reserved for the use of teachers, you could also ask for permission for your child to use this if stairs are a problem.

PE classes, and particularly those which involve strenuous exercises, may be out of the question altogether or might only be possible when your child feels up to them. Make sure that the PE staff are fully aware of your child's condition and of the fact that his or her symptoms may vary considerably from day to day, so that your child is the one who decides whether or not to take part. In other classes, teachers need to understand that your child's concentration may be affected by the condition, particularly on those days when he or she feels overtired, and also that they may need to get up and move around to alleviate joint pain and stiffness. If your child needs extra time to complete homework assignments, such as because of problems which affect the hands and make writing difficult, then again, take this up with the teacher, and if note-taking during lessons is difficult, ask whether handouts can be provided.

Of course, one issue that no-one really likes to think about or consider a possibility is bullying, but unfortunately children can be extremely cruel, especially towards those who are in any way different. A sudden reluctance to attend school, skipping particular classes or a downturn in performance might all be indications that your child is being bullied, so watch out for the signs and discuss it with them should the need arise. Always treat a child's reports of bullying seriously and never advise them to retaliate. Instead, make a note of precisely what happened, when, where and who was involved and report it to the school. Reassure your child that reporting it will not make things worse for them and that the school has an obligation to stamp out bullying behaviour. Under no circumstances should you approach, or allow yourself to be approached by the bully's parents.

Although there will very likely be special considerations which will need to be taken into account in relation to your child's school life, the aim should be to keep things as normal as possible. Children and teenagers typically hate nothing more than being singled out as a special case, so try to get across to teachers the importance of balance.

16

Support for Arthritis Sufferers

Being diagnosed and living with a chronic condition can often be a frightening and alienating experience. Although educating yourself about your condition through books such as this and through talking to your healthcare practitioner can do much to alleviate many of the fears, what many sufferers find especially helpful is to talk to other people who are going through the same feelings and experiencing the same difficulties. Not only does this help them to feel less alone, but those who have lived with the disease for any length of time are typically able to offer invaluable support and advice based on first-hand experience.

Because arthritis is such a common disease in many countries around the world, not only are there some excellent charities which offer their own helplines, but also numerous support groups where sufferers can meet up face to face, as well as online discussion forums where they can stay in touch and exchange thoughts and practical advice. To follow, you will find the details of some of the main resources within the UK and the USA, as well as some of those which are aimed specifically at children and teenagers with arthritis.

Arthritis Support in the UK

Arthritis Care is the largest charity working in support of people with the condition in the UK, and with arthritis sufferers forming its membership as well as directing and being involved in its activities, the support that it offers is based around true understanding. Their website can be found at www.arthritiscare.org.uk, and here you can find contact details for their helpline, as well as links to a variety of other organisations such as the Children's Chronic

Arthritis Association (CCAA). Arthritis Care's online discussion forum, which at the time of writing had almost 15,000 members, can be found at www.arthritiscare.org.uk/forums/ and here you can communicate and share experiences with other sufferers on a whole variety of topics. For details of the support in your local area go to www.arthritiscare.org.uk/InyourArea and click on the area of the map that you are interested in.

The National Rheumatoid Arthritis Society (NRAS) provides information and support specifically for sufferers of this type of the disease, as well as that which is aimed at their families, friends and carers. Their website can be found at www.nras.org.uk/ and if you click on the 'Help for you' tab, you can quickly and easily navigate your way to details of their helpline, details of NRAS groups in your area and various other useful information.

LUPUS UK, is the only national registered charity to support people with systemic lupus erythematosus and discoid lupus – theirwebsite can be found at www.lupusuk.org.uk. The organisation has around 6,000 members and a number of regional groups around the UK which can be found by clicking on 'Regional Group Finder' from the homepage of their website. The organisation also publishes local newsletters and a national magazine with articles and reports relating to the condition.

The National Ankylosing Spondylitis Society (NASS) is dedicated to sufferers of ankylosing spondylitis and their families and its website at www.nass.co.uk offers a comprehensive list of local branches, as well as a members' forum (subject to a membership fee).

In addition to these organisations, Patient.co.uk also lists a number of other charities and support organisations for arthritic and arthritis-related conditions and these can be found at www.patient.co.uk/display/16777259/.

Arthritis Support in the USA

The Arthritis Foundation is the only national not-for profit organisation in the USA to support sufferers of the more than 100 different types of arthritis and related conditions. On the homepage of their website at www.arthritis.org, you just need to insert your ZIP code to find details of your local chapter of the organisation.

Sufferers of psoriatic arthritis and their families, meanwhile, can turn to the Living with Psoriatic Arthritis (PsA) online support group at www.livingwithpsoriaticarthritis.org, which is a dedicated patient-to-patient community for families affected by the disease offering a variety of forum discussions.

The International Scleroderma Network (ISN) available at http://sclero.org/index.html provides a list of support groups for people with scleroderma or you can access the US listings at http://sclero.org/support/swa/listings/support-united-states.html. Simply click on the relevant state and you will find contact details for the support group leaders, as well as a meeting schedule and a link to the area's support group website.

Arthritis sufferers and their families can also find details of meet-up groups around the USA via http://arthritis.meetup.com/.

Support for Younger Sufferers

In addition to offering support for adult sufferers of arthritis, the UK organisation Arthritis Care also offers a free and confidential helpline for young people and their families which is known as The Source. You can find out more details about the service via the link to www.arthritiscare.org.uk/LivingwithArthritis/Young people/Whenyourchildhasarthritis/PublicationsandResources/ Someonetotalkto/Helpline/TheSource. If you want to see what support is available for young people and their families in your area, click on www.arthritiscare.org.uk/LivingwithArthritis/ Youngpeople/Whenyourchildhasarthritis/InyourArea and select the area where you live. Under 25s can also participate in the young people's forum at www.arthritiscare.org.uk/forums/.

Part III

Treating and Managing Arthritis

17

Pain Management

With no definitively identified causes for the various types of arthritis and no known cures, millions of people around the world struggle daily with the pain and other symptoms of these conditions. In fact, during the year 2010, a reported 90% of all calls to the Arthritis Care Helpline were said to be directly related to the pain of arthritis and how to handle it, which serves to illustrate the extent of suffering even after individuals have been diagnosed with and presumably given some treatment for one of these conditions.

The problem with many chronic conditions such as arthritis is that often the pain does not respond fully to the medications which are typically prescribed by GPs. In the same way that the levels and sensations of pain themselves vary enormously from person to person, so too do the effects of the drugs which are intended to control it, with some people experiencing a vast improvement and others seeing very little or even none at all. While some doctors send patients for additional types of treatment, such as physical therapies, others all but give up, and as surgery often is not an option, many sufferers are left to do just that – suffer.

Managing the pain of arthritis, however, is usually not as straightforward as swallowing a few tablets or booking in for a few sessions of physiotherapy. Although these treatments typically do have a part to play in alleviating painful symptoms, often it is only when they are combined with other elements such as exercise, stress management, diet, weight loss, cognitive behavioural therapy, treatment for anxiety and/or depression and education about the condition itself and in relation to coping strategies that they are most effective.

Pain, and especially pain which is experienced over a long period of time, is not just a physical sensation, but rather it affects us on a whole range of different levels, including emotionally, psychologically, socially and occupationally. Trying to treat it at a purely physical level, therefore, only scratches at the surface of the problem, but does not deliver a long-term, all-encompassing solution. In addition, because pain is a totally subjective sensation which is felt differently by every human being, even those who are diagnosed with the same condition and whose physical symptoms suggest the same level of severity, applying the same course of treatment across the board typically does not work either. Instead, treatment needs to be tailored specifically to each individual.

As opposed to the 'standard' approach to treating chronic pain conditions which might involve, for example, a patient being prescribed medications by a GP and seeing a physiotherapist at a local hospital, the concept of pain management applies a multidisciplinary approach from within a facility which is staffed by experts from a whole range of medical backgrounds. A team might therefore comprise pain management consultants, physiotherapists, nurses, occupational therapists, clinical psychologists and dieticians. These specialists work together using their combined skills and knowledge to address all of the factors which might be contributing to the impairment of the patient's quality of life and so, rather than just treating an illness and dealing with discrete symptoms quite separately, it treats the human being as a whole, giving them renewed physical confidence and interrupting the vicious cycle of pain, anxiety and depression.

Chronic pain conditions are complex, and like human beings they cannot be conveniently divided up. Just as we are influenced by physical, emotional and psychological factors, so these same factors influence chronic pain conditions, so that not only physiological damage to our bodies contributes to our experience of pain, but also our past experiences, our attitudes, our state of mind, our levels of stress and our lifestyles. Only when all of these things are taken into account and dealt with simultaneously can a treatment programme provide maximum effect.

Of course, one of the problems with trying to unpick

symptoms and deal with them separately is that you can end up in a situation where, effectively, the left hand has no idea what the right hand is doing. To use a very crude example, a GP who is working separately from a physiotherapist might, for instance, prescribe a drug treatment which helps with one symptom but causes unpleasant or harmful side effects or exacerbates another symptom. Without fully understanding the impact of the drug, the physiotherapist might then adjust his or her treatment regime to take into account the changes in the patient's condition, but in such a way that the therapy then does not have the maximum beneficial effect. When the whole person is treated by a team which is working closely together, however, the various elements of treatment can be constructed and adjusted in such a way as to achieve the very best results.

In the rest of Part III, I will look at some of the main elements which might form part of a pain management programme, starting with some of the most commonly prescribed medications, what they are used for and any potential side effects or contraindications. As I have mentioned, however, it is important to remember that no two treatment programmes are likely to be identical and your own should be put together according to your unique needs and circumstances.

18

Medications and Contraindications

Although the most effective courses of treatment for the various forms of arthritis have been shown time and time again to be those which take a multidisciplinary approach, in many cases both over-the-counter and prescribed medications do play a role in helping to relieve pain and other symptoms, in the early stages at least. While some of these are taken in tablet form, others are administered in the form of injections or applied to the skin in the form of creams and ointments.

The main categories of medications that you are likely to come across, and the ones that you will find covered in this chapter include:

■ Analgesics (painkillers)
■ Non-steroidal anti-inflammatory drugs (NSAIDs)
■ Steroids
■ Muscle relaxants
■ Disease-modifying anti-rheumatic drugs (DMARDs), and
■ Biologic drugs

In some cases only one type of drug might be prescribed, whereas in others a combination will be more appropriate, but either way your doctor or pain management specialist should monitor you carefully to ensure that your medication is having the desired effect and that you are not experiencing any unpleasant or harmful side effects. In addition, before prescribing any medication, he or she should check to see whether you are taking any other types of drug for other conditions. Before purchasing any form of over-the-counter medication, you should also check with your doctor or the pharmacist to ensure that it is suitable to take alongside any other prescription or non-prescription medications that you are already using.

Analgesics

Analgesics, or painkillers as they are more commonly known, work by blocking pain signals or by interfering with the way that the brain interprets those signals, but what they do not do is to have any effect on inflammation. Paracetamol (known as acetaminophen in the USA, Canada, Japan, Hong Kong and one or two other countries) is probably the most widely available and best-known analgesic and, on its own, it is typically used for minor aches and pains and fevers. One of the particular benefits of paracetamol is that it tends to cause far fewer gastrointestinal problems than drugs such as ibuprofen or aspirin, particularly in the elderly, making it the preferred initial choice.

Although paracetamol is generally considered to be a safe drug, like all medications its safety relies entirely on the user taking it in no more than the recommended doses. If used long term, if single or multiple overdoses are taken or if the drug is taken in association with alcohol, it can lead to liver damage and possibly to fatal consequences. Perhaps one of the greatest dangers with paracetamol comes with accidental overdose, because the drug is contained in hundreds of over-the-counter cold and flu remedies, cough medicines and treatments for sinus problems for example.

Because long-term or inappropriate use of paracetamol can itself cause liver damage, anyone with a pre-existing liver disease should not use it and it should also be avoided by those with an allergy to the drug. In the case of alcoholics and pregnant and breast-feeding women, meanwhile, it should only be used with caution, and women in the first trimester of pregnancy are advised to avoid it altogether. Those who use anticoagulant and certain other types of medications should only take paracetamol under the direction of their doctors as it can increase the effects of these drugs or the harmful effects on the liver. Another thing which is worth mentioning in relation to paracetamol which is particularly relevant to those who suffer from gout and diabetes is that the drug can interfere with the results of laboratory tests which are used to check levels of uric acid and blood glucose.

Although paracetamol rarely gives rise to any serious side effects, itchiness of the skin and a rash do occasionally occur. Used over a long period, meanwhile, it can cause toxic hepatitis, with initial symptoms of nausea, vomiting and sweating.

Alongside paracetamol, another group of painkillers includes the opiate and opioid drugs. Opiates are derived directly from the opium poppy, whereas opioids are synthetic drugs which are designed to emulate opium, and typically these drugs are used for moderate to severe pain. In the UK and some other countries, opioids such as codeine and dihydrocodeine are combined with paracetamol, aspirin or ibuprofen and sold as over-the-counter medications such as Co-Dydramol (paracetamol and dihydrocodeine). Other stronger opioids, meanwhile, are only available on prescription.

One of the greatest dangers of the opiate and opioid drugs is that they carry the risk of physical dependence, which means that stopping the medication suddenly can lead to unpleasant withdrawal symptoms. In terms of the side effects, meanwhile, the most common ones include drowsiness, a dry mouth, nausea, vomiting, itching of the skin and constipation. Opioids can also cause depression in some of those who use them, as well as changes to libido and erectile dysfunction and they may not be suitable for use by those with respiratory problems or nursing mothers.

Of course, tablets are not the only form of painkiller available today, and some people with arthritis find analgesic patches to be very effective. These patches, which contain a painkilling drug, are placed on to the skin directly over the site of the pain and the drug is released through the skin and into the bloodstream over a period of time. In addition, there are also topical lotions and creams, such as those containing capsaicin (the active ingredient in chilli peppers) which can provide effective pain relief when rubbed into the skin around the painful area.

Non-steroidal Anti-inflammatory Drugs

Unlike analgesics, which only act to relieve pain but do not help to alleviate inflammation, non-steroidal anti-inflammatory drugs (NSAIDs) work to alleviate both and they are the most commonly prescribed drugs for patients with arthritis. Some of the most common NSAIDs include ibuprofen, which is sold under a variety of brand names such as Nurofen and Advil, aspirin, naproxen (brand names include Naprosyn, Anaprox and Aleve), nabumetone, which is sold as Relafen, and diclofenac, which is probably most often seen as Voltaren or Voltarol. At lower doses, NSAIDs are sold as over-the-counter medications, but higher doses are available on prescription only.

NSAIDs work by blocking the chemicals in the blood (prostaglandins) which promote inflammation, pain, muscle cramps and fever. These prostaglandins are produced within the body's cells by the enzyme known as cyclooxygenase (COX), which comes in two forms, COX-1 and COX-2. The more traditional types of NSAIDs block both of these enzymes, but in strongly inhibiting COX-1, they can have a tendency to promote ulcers, stomach upsets and gastrointestinal bleeding and the risk of these side effects increases significantly with age. Having said this, however, side effects can be minimised by taking the medication with or after meals, restricting alcohol intake and by not smoking.

Traditional NSAIDs are contraindicated for anyone who:

- Is allergic to aspirin or any NSAID. An allergic reaction is characterised by rash, swelling of the face and sometimes breathing difficulties and anyone experiencing these symptoms should seek immediate medical attention
- Has a history of peptic ulcers
- Suffers from a defect of the blood clotting system
- Is currently taking anticoagulant medication, or
- Is pregnant or breast-feeding

As concerns have been raised relating to the potential of traditional NSAIDs and COX-2 inhibitors to increase the risk of cardiovascular problems, especially in those who have a history of heart disease or stroke, the current medical advice is that these people should also avoid the use of these medications. Anyone with asthma or impairment of the kidneys or liver, meanwhile, should only take NSAIDs under strict medical supervision.

Because of the potential problems with NSAIDs which act strongly on the COX-1 enzyme, a newer form of anti-inflammatory drugs known as COX-2 inhibitors has more recently been developed. Medications such as Celebrex, which have little effect on the COX-1 enzyme, present a much lower risk of internal bleeding and ulcers than traditional NSAIDs. However, they are contraindicated for those who are allergic to celecoxib or any of the other ingredients, people who have experienced asthma or hives, those who are allergic to aspirin or any other type of traditional NSAID and women in late pregnancy.

For those suffering from gout, aspirin should be avoided as this can increase the levels of uric acid in the blood. The only exception to this might be in the case of low-dose aspirin which is prescribed to protect against heart disease or similar conditions, but once again, this should only be taken if specifically advised by a qualified doctor.

As with analgesics, there are alternatives to anti-inflammatory medications which are taken orally; lotions, gels and patches containing anti-inflammatory medications are also in use by some arthritis sufferers.

Corticosteroids

Corticosteroids, or steroids as they are more commonly known, are like the 'big guns' in terms of treating inflammation. In autoimmune disorders they work by suppressing the immune system, blocking the production of the substances which trigger inflammation, so that healthy tissues incur less damage as a result of the underlying immune system dysfunction. They may be used in certain cases involving rheumatoid, psoriatic and reactive arthritis, as well as to alleviate pain and inflammation in systemic lupus erythematosus, polymyalgia rheumatica, ankylosing spondylitis and scleroderma. In addition, they may be prescribed for other conditions which are sometimes associated with arthritis, such as vasculitis and Sjögren's syndrome.

Although corticosteroids are typically very effective at treating inflammation, not to mention being fast-acting, and may at times be administered in high doses, generally doctors will try to reduce oral dosages as soon as possible because of the fact that they can cause a range of side effects, some of which can be quite serious. The most common ones, however, include:

■ High blood pressure
■ Increased appetite and weight gain
■ Swelling or puffiness of the face
■ Water retention
■ Decreased resistance to infections
■ Muscle weakness
■ Irritation of the stomach
■ Increased growth of body hair
■ Blurring of vision
■ Cataracts or glaucoma
■ Sleep problems
■ Sudden mood swings
■ Nervousness and restlessness
■ A tendency to bruise easily
■ In diabetics, a worsening of the condition

In addition, one of the considerable downsides of steroids is that they can also increase the likelihood of osteoporosis, in which the bones become thinner and more brittle.

The recommended dosage of steroids varies according to the patient, the type of steroid and the strength of the drug. As I have mentioned, higher doses may be prescribed in the case of dangerous flares of inflammation, although often this is just a temporary measure until other slower-acting medications start to take effect. At lower doses, they may be used to reduce the likelihood of flares and to protect, not only joints, but also the eyes and the internal organs from inflammation. Whatever the dose, however, it is important that the use of steroids not be discontinued suddenly. This is because the drug mimics the effect of the naturally produced hormone cortisol, and gradual reduction in dose allows the adrenal glands to resume natural cortisol production.

As well as being administered orally, corticosteroids are also given by injection, and the benefit here is that the drug is delivered directly to the site of the inflammation. In some cases this might mean injecting directly into the joint, whereas in others it might be into an inflamed area nearby. In the case of a disease such as rheumatoid arthritis in which there is often considerable inflammation in the joints, steroid injections might be administered on a fairly regular basis, but because they act in only a localised area of the body, there is a much lower risk of side effects. Sometimes there might be a flare in joint pain within the first 24 hours after the injection has been given and, as with any injection, there is a small chance of infection being introduced into the joint, but other than that, thinning of the skin or a change in the colour of the skin around the injection site, facial flushing and changes to the menstrual cycle are the only other occasional side effects to be experienced.

Of course, how long the effects of a steroid injection last will depend on whether the drug used is of the shorter or longer-acting variety. Short-acting steroids, which normally provide effective relief within just hours, usually last at least a week, whereas the longer-acting drugs may last for two months or more, but typically take several days before they become effective. In some cases, a local anaesthetic is given at the same time as the steroid injection, in which case there is immediate, albeit only temporary pain relief.

Muscle Relaxants

Although regularly used in the treatment of fibromyalgia to help with the painful muscle spasms which are typically experienced as part of the condition, as well as to improve the quality of sleep, muscle relaxants are less often used in the treatment of arthritis. The exception to this might be if pain is caused by the straining of the muscles to support joints which are affected by osteoarthritis and other forms of the disease.

The types of muscle relaxants which are used to help relieve muscular pain, as opposed to the types which are used during surgery to effectively paralyse the patient and stop involuntary muscle movement, act on the central nervous system. They do, however, typically cause a number of unpleasant side effects, including drowsiness, impaired movement, impaired sense of coordination and, in some cases, a high risk of dependence. Particularly in older sufferers of osteoarthritis, the side effects often outweigh the benefits of the medication.

Disease-modifying Anti-rheumatic Drugs

Disease-modifying anti-rheumatic drugs (DMARDs), rather than being used to treat the specific symptoms of certain types of arthritis, are designed to actually alter the course of the disease. Although they are most commonly used in the treatment of rheumatoid arthritis, some types are also prescribed for sufferers of psoriatic arthritis, ankylosing spondylitis, systemic lupus erythematosus and juvenile idiopathic arthritis.

The way that DMARDs work is by suppressing the immune system so that the progression of the disease is slowed down and so that the amount of damage is limited. Because inflammation in the joints can cause permanent damage, and because some DMARDs can take up to three or four months to take effect, it is important that these drugs are prescribed as soon after diagnosis as possible. In the intervening period before the effects become noticeable to the patient, doctors will often prescribe NSAIDs or corticosteroids to help with pain and inflammation.

The main types of DMARD to be prescribed for arthritis include:

- Methotrexate (brand names include Rheumatrex and Trexall)
- Sulfasalazine (Azulfidine, Sulfazine)
- Azathioprine (Imuran, Azasan)
- Cyclosporine (Neoral, Sandimmune, Gengraf)
- Cyclophosphamide (Cytoxan, Neosar)
- Hydroxychloroquine (Plaquenil, Quineprox)
- Leflunomide (Arava), and
- Gold injections

Originally used as a chemotherapy treatment for cancer, methotrexate is one of the most commonly prescribed DMARDs for arthritis, although it is used at much lower doses for this purpose. Patients who take the drug, however, do need to be carefully monitored as it can cause a range of potentially serious side effects, including:

- Stomach upsets
- Soreness of the mouth
- Interference with the ability of the bone marrow to produce blood cells and consequential fevers, infections, swollen lymph nodes and bleeding
- Liver damage (alcohol should be avoided if possible when taking methotrexate)
- Lung damage and shortness of breath
- Birth defects

On the plus side, however, methotrexate is normally safe to take for long periods of time, can even be taken by children and tends to be very effective in terms of slowing down the progression of arthritis. In addition, the risk of certain side effects can be reduced by taking regular daily or weekly doses of folic acid. Regular blood testing is recommended during the course of treatment though, to ensure that the drug is not having any adverse effects.

Biologic Drugs

Other newer types of drug which are being used in the treatment of rheumatoid arthritis, especially in cases where the patient has not responded to other disease-modifying drugs, are biologic drugs, which are sometimes also referred to as tumour necrosis factor (TNF) inhibitors. Often combined with DMARDs, these drugs block the immune system's signals which lead to joint damage and can be very effective at controlling inflammation.

TNF inhibitors are either injected under the skin or administered directly into a vein and often they can be self-administered at home. Some of the more common drugs include adalimumab (brand name Humira), etanercept (Enbrel) and infliximab (Remicade). Like other drugs these too can cause side effects, but typically these are fewer than in the case of other DMARDs. Patients may, for example, experience severe infections or adverse effects on liver or blood counts and TNF inhibitors should only be used with extreme caution to treat patients with weak hearts. Because these drugs are relatively new, however, it could be many years before other long-term side effects begin to show themselves.

In addition to TNF inhibitors, other new biologic drugs which are designed to target the specific parts of the immune system which give rise to inflammation are beginning to find their way on to the market. Rituximab, which is sold under the brand name of Rituxan, is one such drug which may be prescribed if other TNF inhibitors are found to be ineffective. This particular medication is normally administered by infusion in hospital, with two infusions being given two weeks apart, usually once or twice per year.

Other Drugs

Alongside the wide variety of drugs which are prescribed for a number of different types of arthritis, there are also other medications which are specific to particular forms of the disease. As discussed under the heading of Gout in Chapter 3 for example, colchicine is a drug which is used to stop the migration of white blood cells into the site of uric acid crystals, so inhibiting the release of lactic acid and pro-inflammatory enzymes which cause the pain and swelling characteristic of the condition. Depending upon the type of arthritis that you are diagnosed with, therefore, you may be offered other different types of drugs which have not been discussed in this book. Should this be the case, do not hesitate to ask your doctor how the medication is designed to help you, as well as checking out any potential side effects. In addition, of course, with ongoing research into the various forms of arthritis, new drugs will continue to come on to the market.

Care and Use of Medications

As I mentioned earlier, all drugs have the potential to cause side effects in some people and almost without exception they can be extremely dangerous if taken in excessive doses. Using and caring for your medications appropriately is therefore vital to keep you and your family safe and to ensure that you receive maximum benefit from them. Here are a few tips to bear in mind.

1. Take your medications at the same times of the day so that you do not forget and try to associate them with regular daily activities such as brushing your teeth in the morning or watching the 6 o'clock news. If they need to be taken with food, then lay them out ready at mealtimes when you set out the cutlery.

2. Although there are pill boxes available which allow you to set out different tablets for different times of day or days of the week and which are intended to make it easier to see whether or not you are up-to-date with your medications, the old advice of keeping your tablets in their original bottles or packages still stands. Not only does doing so mean that you have the correct labels with the correct instructions to hand, but also in the case of emergency, it is easier for other people, including medical staff, to see instantly which drugs you are taking. Another reason why this is particularly important is that many drugs are supplied in bottles with child-proof caps, whereas other types of pill boxes are typically very easy to open.

3. Never reduce the prescribed dosage of medication or stop taking it without first consulting with your doctor. Not only could this cause your arthritis symptoms to worsen, but as explained under the heading of Corticosteroids, it can also have other detrimental effects on the body's systems.

4. Always make sure that you have sufficient stocks of your medication so that you do not run out.

5. Never take more than the prescribed dosage as this could have extremely serious consequences.

6. Crushing or breaking some tablets can impact on their effectiveness, so always try to take them in their whole form.

7. Always keep your medications out of the reach of children.

A Note about Cannabis

Much is publicised about the pain-relieving effects of cannabis, but while attitudes towards it may appear to have become more relaxed over the years, it is still, nevertheless, an illegal drug in the UK and most states in the USA. In addition to this, some studies have shown that long-term use of cannabis can bring about mental deterioration, as well as changes to personality and behaviour. For arthritis sufferers whose mobility may already be affected by the disease, being under the influence of cannabis may also put them at greater risk of falls. Finally, cannabis may have an adverse reaction with other medications that you are taking for your arthritis and could possibly cause unpleasant or even dangerous side effects.

Non-Pharmaceutical Treatments

Alongside the wide variety of pharmaceutical treatments which are available to help relieve the symptoms of arthritis and, in some cases, to slow down the progression of the disease, non-pharmaceutical treatments can also play an enormous role in helping to manage the condition as part of a multidisciplinary approach. Not only do these treatments help to improve mobility, strength and flexibility, but they also contribute greatly to the alleviation of pain and help to ensure increased levels of independence and a vastly improved overall quality of life.

Physiotherapy

People who suffer from arthritis typically find themselves in a Catch 22 situation. Not only the pain and stiffness caused by their condition, but also the fear of causing greater damage to the affected joints discourages them from exercising and taking part in their normal daily activities and sometimes causes them to alter their gait and posture to compensate for painful joints. As a consequence, levels of pain and stiffness increase, leading to even greater immobility, and muscles begin to lose their strength. In some cases, compensatory movements also put strain on other muscles in the body, creating further areas of pain. All of this, of course, makes the sufferer even less inclined to take part in any form of exercise and so the vicious cycle continues.

Exercise plays an extremely important role in the management of arthritis and in some cases the benefits derived from it can even mean that patients are able to stop taking pharmaceutical medications altogether. It is vital, however, to understand precisely which exercises to carry out and how to do so safely, and this is where the role of the physiotherapist comes in.

Physiotherapists are professional practitioners who are trained in anatomy, physiology and the concepts of movement. They work with their patients to design tailored exercise programmes which are specific to their needs, and the types of exercises that they recommend depend entirely on the type of arthritis, the severity of the condition and the patient's age and overall state of health. They use their clinical judgement to assess the patient's condition, devise a programme of simple exercises which are taught to the patient so that he or she is able to continue with them at home and then continue to review the patient's progress for as long as is necessary. The physiotherapists that you will find in pain management clinics work directly alongside the multidisciplinary team of specialists who are jointly responsible for your care, including the pain management consultant, nurses, occupational therapists and clinical psychologists.

The exercise plans which are devised by physiotherapists on behalf of arthritis patients are designed to achieve a number of aims. Firstly, they help to eliminate stiffness and to improve and maintain joint mobility and range of motion without putting undue stress on the joints. Secondly, they promote the strengthening of muscles, as stronger muscles help to stabilise weakened joints. Finally, they help with weight reduction, as well as building stamina and endurance and addressing any examples of poor posture which might be contributing to pain and discomfort. Not only will a trained physiotherapist teach you the exercises that you need to perform to achieve these goals, but also how to prepare yourself for exercising, such as by warming up your muscles, in order to avoid any further damage. In addition, they will show you how to use heat and cold therapies safely at home to help alleviate pain and inflammation.

Physiotherapists do not only help patients through exercise, however, but also through a range of other physical therapies, such as manipulation and massage, which are again aimed at increasing mobility and alleviating pain. I will look at some of these other therapies under the heading of Complementary Therapies further on in this chapter. In addition, physiotherapists provide advice and assistance on the use of walking aids such as sticks, crutches and walking frames should these be necessary.

Of course, unlike some of the pharmaceutical treatments which are taken orally or given by injection, exercise does not usually provide instant results. For this reason, it is not uncommon for patients to give physical therapy less attention than it deserves or even to give up with exercises altogether within a short space of time. This, however, is a huge mistake and typically causes patients to endure unnecessary suffering and a continual deterioration in their quality of life. Those who persevere, on the other hand, often find that they are able to enjoy a much more active and comfortable existence.

Choosing a properly trained and qualified physiotherapist is absolutely vital, not only to ensure that you gain maximum benefit from your treatment, but also to ensure your safety. Always be sure to check out the qualifications of any physiotherapist that you are considering using, but also remember that a joined-up and holistic approach to treatment has been shown to be far more effective.

Occupational Therapy

Although there is some crossover between physiotherapy and occupational therapy, the former is more concerned with evaluating, improving and maintaining the physical functions of the body by reducing pain and inflammation, improving the range of motion of the joints and helping patients to walk independently or with the use of walking aids, whereas the latter concentrates on improving a person's capabilities in terms of carrying out his or her normal daily activities at work and at home with minimal disruption. For many people, occupational therapy is a vital part of treatment in terms of allowing them to maintain their independence.

As with physiotherapy, the first aim of occupational therapy is to assess the patient's current capabilities and needs. You may, for example, experience difficulties with dressing yourself or carrying out household chores such as cooking, struggle with transport issues or have functional problems which relate to your paid occupation. Once these needs and issues have been established, the therapist will then use his or her skills and experience to suggest ways to make your life easier and more manageable.

Along with providing recommendations for different ways of doing things which will help to protect your joints, one of the key roles of the occupational therapist is to make you aware of the range of tools, gadgets and adaptations which might help you to carry out your daily activities more safely and easily. These might include anything from simple pieces of kitchen equipment such as kettle tippers or ergonomically designed cutlery to adaptations to the home such as the installation of a stair lift. In addition, your occupational therapist should be able to advise you on the use of splints to support and protect the joints which are affected by arthritis and may be able to provide these for you, as well as showing you how to carry out movements in such a way that you do not cause any further damage. In some cases, the therapist may even be able to visit your home to carry out an assessment and determine whether any alterations or adaptations might be beneficial and help you to retain your independence.

Podiatry

Podiatry, or chiropody as it is more commonly known, is the branch of medicine which is devoted to the care of the feet, ankles and lower legs. Because different forms of arthritis can frequently affect the feet, making both walking and standing particularly painful or uncomfortable, the role of the podiatrist can often be a significant one. As trained and qualified practitioners, podiatrists understand how inflammation and joint degeneration affects the feet, ankles and lower legs and they are able to recommend courses of action or specialised footwear or insoles to make walking easier, safer and more comfortable.

When you visit a podiatrist, the first thing that he or she will do will be to examine the way that you walk, paying particular attention to such things as your range of motion, the pressure which is placed on each of the feet and the way in which you compensate for painful foot and leg joints. The specialist may also recommend X-rays or scans to get a clearer picture of the bones and joints which are affected in order to be able to make the best possible recommendations to alleviate your pain and discomfort. Should specialised footwear be required, the podiatrist will take whatever measurements are necessary and then arrange a follow-up visit for a fitting and any further appointments which might be necessary to monitor your progress.

Complementary Therapies

The range of complementary or alternative therapies available today is vast and includes everything from ancient techniques such as acupuncture and yoga to more modern pain-relieving solutions such as transcutaneous electrical nerve stimulation (TENS). Although more and more people are finding these complementary therapies to be extremely effective in the long-term management of arthritis, it has to be said that older sufferers in particular can often be somewhat wary of trying them out despite a great deal of evidence in support of their benefits.

Of course, like the more traditional forms of arthritis treatment such as pharmaceutical medications and physiotherapy, complementary therapies do not provide a cure for the condition, but they can help greatly to ease the pain and some of the other symptoms of arthritis and they are often used alongside more conventional treatments. In this section, therefore, I will take a look at some of the most popular complementary therapies and precisely what they involve.

Acupuncture

The ancient Chinese healing practice of acupuncture has been around for around 2,000 years and, although it does have its sceptics, it is still proving to be a highly effective method of pain relief for a great many people suffering from a wide range of conditions involving pain. Not only this though, but scientific research carried out in recent years has demonstrated that it really does work. One study which was conducted by the US National Institutes of Health on a group of patients suffering from arthritis of the knee, for example, showed that acupuncture patients experienced a 40% decrease in pain levels and almost the same level of improvement in joint function, and other studies have shown similarly favourable results in sufferers of rheumatoid arthritis.

The practice of acupuncture involves inserting ultra-fine, sterile needles into strategic parts of the body. Although it is not fully understood quite how this works to alleviate pain, the ancient belief is that when the flow of life energy (known as qi and pronounced 'chee') becomes blocked or out of balance, this leads to pain or illness, and that stimulating these points of blockage via the insertion of needles into the skin helps to unblock or correct the flow. Whether you happen to concur with these beliefs, however, is immaterial, and indeed many a disbeliever has achieved at least temporary relief from chronic pain through acupuncture.

Alexander Technique

The Alexander Technique is a method for becoming more aware of the body and how it moves and of changing movement habits with a view to removing muscle tension. It is aimed at improving ease and freedom of movement, as well as balance, support and co-ordination. By re-educating mind and body, it teaches individuals how to use the appropriate amount of energy for a particular activity so that they have more energy to go around, as well as how to improve posture and so alleviate pain.

The Alexander Technique is usually taught by qualified Alexander teachers who advise on posture and patterns of movement.

Hydrotherapy

Hydrotherapy has been a popular method of alleviating pain and maintaining good health since Roman times. Essentially it involves the use of water, either internally or externally, to:

- Improve circulation so that the cells and tissues of the body are kept well-supplied with oxygen and nourishment
- Stimulate the release of endorphins, the body's natural pain-relieving and mood-enhancing hormones
- Provide effective stress relief
- Detoxify the body to encourage a stronger immune system

In relation to arthritis, hydrotherapy might take the form of the use of heat or cold packs which are applied to the area of pain or inflammation, or taking part in special exercises in a warm-water pool. Many arthritis sufferers find this latter form of treatment to be particularly beneficial because the warm water helps to soothe and relax the muscles and ease joint pain, while of course the water supports the weight of the body so that the joints are not under as much pressure as they would be on dry land. Because hydrotherapy exercises are typically less painful to carry out, many people find that they can do more and that they are easier to stick with than conventional forms of exercise.

Osteopathy

Osteopathy is a treatment which involves the gentle stretching, massage and manipulation of joints and muscles and its aim is to ensure good structural balance in the body.

When you visit an osteopath, one of the first things that will happen is that he or she will take your full medical history in order to make an assessment of your condition and the most appropriate form of treatment. The specialist will also look at your posture and at how you move your body, taking careful note of when and where you experience pain, as well as using touch to determine areas of sensitivity and tension.

Of course, the type of technique which is used by the osteopath will vary according to his or her findings, and will also take into account the nature of your condition, your age and your general levels of fitness. Typically though, they might include different types of massage, as well as muscle stretching and joint mobilisation. As some of the techniques used in osteopathy can be quite rigorous, it is absolutely vital to choose a practitioner who is fully trained and qualified, as well as one who is experienced in treating patients with arthritis.

Homeopathy

Homeopathy is a treatment process which has been around since the 18th century and which is still considered by many laymen and medical practitioners to be fairly controversial. Basically, it works on the theory that 'like cures like' and it involves using minute amounts of natural substances to trigger the body's own natural defences against specific symptoms. Research into homeopathy has shown conflicting results, but still some people who have tried it have experienced excellent results.

As I have said, the natural substances which are used to prepare homeopathic remedies are usually only used in tiny amounts, which in some cases amount to no more than one part per million. Nevertheless, as some of these substances are highly poisonous if taken in larger quantities, it is extremely important that anyone considering homeopathy as an alternative treatment chooses a qualified practitioner to work with.

Yoga

When most of us think of yoga what comes to mind is people tying themselves up in knots, which for an arthritis sufferer almost certainly does not sound like a very sensible or even possible thing to do. The physical movements in yoga, however, are slow and controlled and so can provide a gentle form of exercise which helps to ease pain and stiff joints and relax muscles, whilst at the same time increasing flexibility, improving muscle strength and stamina and promoting balance.

Yoga though, goes further than just merely addressing the physical aspects of arthritis, because of course this ancient practice has important psychological benefits too. It is a spiritual practice which many people find particularly helpful in terms of restoring emotional balance and enhancing mental well-being and its effects often lead to anxiety, stress and other negative feelings being replaced with a more positive energy.

Although yoga is generally safe for arthritis sufferers, as with any form of exercise, it is wise to check with your healthcare practitioner before signing up for a yoga class just to make sure that there are no physical limitations or restrictions that you should be observing.

Transcutaneous Electrical Nerve Stimulation (TENS)

A far cry from some of the ancient arts and practices that I have discussed so far, transcutaneous electrical nerve stimulation (TENS) is a method of sending low-intensity electrical impulses to certain parts of the body. When used at a high frequency, a TENS machine sends messages to the brain which block pain signals, whereas at a lower frequency it is thought to stimulate the production of the body's natural pain-relieving hormones, endorphins.

TENS machines are used by people all around the world as a form of pain relief, but many people will associate their use with the pain of childbirth. Nowadays, not only are they still used regularly for this purpose, but also by women of all ages to deal with menstrual pain and cramping. For arthritis sufferers though, they seem to have variable results, with some experiencing little or no effect and others gaining either shorter or longer-term pain relief.

The TENS machine itself is a lightweight, battery operated device which is small enough to fit in the palm of the hand. It has leads running from the main unit with either two or four rubber electrodes connected to the ends and these electrodes are either self-adhesive or attach to the skin (usually on either side of the area where you are experiencing most pain) using an adhesive tape or a water-based gel. Once the electrodes are attached, the user can then control the current using a dial. At a low voltage current there is normally a tingling or buzzing sensation, and at a higher voltage the sensation should be strong, but not so strong as to cause pain or discomfort. The machine can be used as often as every alternate hour throughout the course of the day as required.

Although TENS is not suitable for use by anyone who is fitted with a pacemaker or any other kind of electrical device, or by women who are in the early stages of pregnancy, they can be used safely by most people. Do check with your healthcare provider beforehand, however, just to ensure that it is appropriate for your use.

The complementary therapies which I have outlined in this section are all widely available nowadays, but one very important thing to remember is that not all of these disciplines are subject to any form of regulation and so basically anyone can set themselves up in business as a practitioner. In some cases, those who offer complementary therapies may not hold any relevant qualifications and may have received little or no training in the area in which they purport to be experts. Some even go so far as to make extravagant but scientifically unsupported claims as to the effectiveness of a particular treatment or recommend that patients curtail the use of prescribed medications or other treatments recommended by qualified doctors, which can of course be extremely dangerous.

If you are interested in trying one or more complementary therapies, always check out the credentials of the service provider carefully in advance or, better still, take advice from your pain management specialist and only use those services which he or she provides directly or recommends.

Surgery

Although most people with arthritis are unlikely to need surgery, as we saw in Chapter 3, there are occasions when joints can become so damaged or when other treatments fail to bring about any beneficial effect that it may become the most appropriate option.

There are various types of surgery which might be performed to help patients with arthritis, such as:

- Arthroscopy – a minimally invasive procedure which is typically used to repair damaged tendons and ligaments or to remove loose bone and cartilage
- Osteotomy – an operation in which bone is cut in order to help realign it and so reduce deformity
- Fusion – a surgical procedure which is aimed at making the bones more stable and is most commonly carried out on the bones in the spine (the spinal vertebrae). Two or more bones may be fused together using screw fixings and bone grafting may also be necessary
- Arthroplasty – in which a damaged joint is replaced with an artificial one. The most common joint replacements are those involving the knees and hips, but ankle, wrist, finger, elbow and shoulder joints can also be replaced

Although surgery can sometimes be the only viable option to deal with severely damaged joints and the results typically lead to a great reduction in pain levels or the complete alleviation of symptoms, all surgery involves at least some degree of risk and in some cases the operation can fail, which means that a further operation may be required. In elderly people in particular, as well as those who suffer from additional illnesses such as heart disease, the risk of surgery needs to be weighed against the potential benefit which might be gained.

As I mentioned earlier in this book, because of the cost of joint replacements and the fact that the number of these operations has spiralled in recent years, many UK authorities have placed strict criteria which have to be met before an individual can be considered for surgery. Because excessive pressure on the larger weight-bearing joints such as the knees and the hips can cause damage to the joints, one of the most significant factors to be taken into consideration is the patient's weight, and those who fail to achieve the prescribed weight limits may not be eligible for surgery.

Herbal Remedies and Supplements

Herbal treatments, like homeopathy, are another area of controversy in relation to arthritis. Although there are a great many companies which advertise herbal treatments specifically for the purpose of relieving arthritis symptoms, a report which was issued by the Arthritis Research Campaign (now known as Arthritis Research UK) in 2009 showed that most have very little or no effect on the two most common forms of the disease, namely osteoarthritis and rheumatoid arthritis. The only four real exceptions to this were:

- Fish oils extracted from oily fish such as salmon, mackerel and sardines scored a maximum of 5 out of 5 for effectiveness in relation to rheumatoid arthritis, as well as getting a 'green light' for safety
- Capsaicin gel scored 5 out of 5 for effectiveness
- Phytodolor, a herbal medicine which is based on extracts of aspen, golden rod and common ash, and the nutritional supplement S adenosyl-L-methionine (SAMe) both received 4 out of 5 for osteoarthritis

The following, meanwhile, were shown to have little or no effect on rheumatoid arthritis:

- Antler velvet
- Blackcurrant seed oil
- Collagen
- Eazmov herbal preparation
- Feverfew
- Flaxseed oil
- Green-lipped mussels
- Homeopathy
- Reumalex herbal mixture
- Selenium
- Tong luo kai bi Chinese herb
- Vitamins A, C and E anti-oxidant vitamins
- Willow bark

For osteoarthritis, glucosamine, which is one of the most widely-taken products, proved to be more effective in the form of glucosamine sulphate than glucosamine hydrochloride.

As far as safety is concerned, a quarter of the compounds which were included in the report were awarded an 'amber' safety classification, meaning that important side effects had been reported. The Chinese herbal medicine which is known as 'thunder god vine', meanwhile was given a 'red' safety classification and was found to have serious side effects including nausea and hair loss.

With any herbal treatment, it is important to remember that even though they are made from natural substances, they can sometimes cause serious side effects in just the same way as pharmaceutical medications and some are positively contraindicated for those with certain other conditions, as well as for children and pregnant women.

As far as dietary supplements such as vitamins and minerals are concerned, always remember that, as the name suggests, these are intended to supplement rather than replace a good, healthy diet.

Advice for Dealing with Specialists

Whether you choose to work alongside your GP and a range of other separate practitioners to treat and manage your arthritis, or whether placing your care in the hands of a team of pain management specialists is your preferred option, it is important that you feel confident in your healthcare providers and that you get the best out of your appointments with them. Here are a few tips to help you achieve both of these ends.

1. Before each of your appointments, write down the things that you want to raise so that you do not forget anything important. Also, prioritise your list so that the most important things are dealt with first.
2. Whether in relation to your condition, your treatment or anything else, never pretend that you understand something if you do not. At the very least this can lead to disappointment if your expectations are not met, and at worst it could be dangerous, particularly if what you have not understood relates to your medications or whether it is safe to take part in certain activities. Always ask for a more detailed or simpler explanation if something is not clear. Taking notes during your consultation can help to avoid any confusion later on, especially if there is a lot of information to take in.
3. Make sure that you are absolutely certain in terms of medications. Ask your doctor why you need to take them, how they work, what dosage you need to take and how often, how long you need to take the drugs for, what the potential side effects are and under what circumstances you might need to seek immediate medical advice or assistance should you experience side effects.
4. If you feel that any aspect of your treatment does not suit you or is causing additional problems, such as side effects from medications, always be sure to tell your doctor.
5. Certain subjects might feel quite embarrassing to raise, such as sexual problems caused by medications or symptoms which affect certain areas of the body. However delicate the issue though, always raise it with your doctor as it may be a matter of some significance and it will almost certainly be something that he or she can help

you with. Remember, there is probably nothing that you could tell your doctor that he or she has not heard hundreds of times before.

6. If you do not feel comfortable attending your appointments alone or you think that you might forget important details of what has been discussed, then take a relative or friend along with you. Even if they have to wait outside while certain examinations are carried out, they should be able to be with you throughout most of the consultation.

7. If you are in any way unhappy about the way that you have been treated by your healthcare provider or about the information or the treatment you are being given, then raise the issue with your consultant. Never just sit on your concerns as they will only cause you additional stress.

The Role of Cognitive Behavioural Therapy

As I mentioned back in Chapter 9, chronic pain conditions are complex and not only do they affect sufferers at a physical level, but they also have the very real potential to affect them emotionally, psychologically and behaviourally too. Diseases such as arthritis which have no cure and can ultimately only be managed can impact enormously on the lives of patients, leaving them feeling unable to cope on an indefinite basis. The way that we think and behave in the face of such illnesses, however, can do a great deal to influence the experience of pain, making it either better or worse.

Something which is quite common in people with arthritis and other types of chronic pain conditions is that they tend to focus all of their attention on the disease to the exclusion of the good and positive things in their lives. Essentially, the disease takes over and starts to control the sufferer, and as negativity sets in and everything begins to feel hopeless, so every aspect of the person's life starts to spiral downwards. Cognitive behavioural therapy, or CBT as it is known for short, is a form of therapy which is aimed at changing attitudes and the behaviours which stem from them so that patients feel empowered to live happy and successful lives in spite of their illness.

Now, before I go on to look at precisely how CBT works, there are three things which are probably worth mentioning at this stage. First of all, the mere mention of the words 'psychological' and 'therapy' within the space of a couple of paragraphs may have some readers feeling slightly uneasy, but it is important to understand that CBT is quite unlike other forms of psychotherapy which are aimed at dealing with deep-rooted past experiences. In fact, its purpose is to deal very much with the here and now and to provide patients with practical tools to help them cope better with their everyday lives.

The second thing to know is that you may well hear about CBT in relation to other areas other than chronic pain conditions, and that is because it is used in the treatment of a whole range of different issues, including things like trauma, bereavement, obsessive compulsive disorders, eating disorders, drug and alcohol abuse, anger management problems and anxiety and depression. Just because it can be applied to all of these areas, however, in no way suggests that you are suffering from some kind of mental problem, because CBT is also used extremely successfully in the treatment of cancer patients and others with potentially fatal illnesses. Clearly the areas that CBT is used to address are very different in the case of each of these examples, but the underlying principles of the treatment and the techniques used do remain the same. The simple fact is that everyone, and I do mean everyone without exception, can benefit from CBT. It is just that only when individuals face particular difficulties in life does it tend to be offered to them or do they seek it out for themselves.

My final point about CBT before I go on is that this particular form of therapy has been the subject of considerable research in relation to chronic pain conditions during the past couple of decades and has been proved time and time again to improve, not only psychological function, but physical function too. Studies have consistently shown that when patients' attitudes towards their illness are adjusted and they are able to see things in a more positive light, and when they learn new and more productive ways of coping with their illness, they feel the benefits in a physical sense and record considerable reductions in pain and other symptoms.

So, with those issues out of the way, precisely how is CBT applied to patients who are suffering from chronic arthritis? Well, one of the first aims of the treatment is for patients to learn about the ways in which chronic pain can affect our thoughts, perceptions and reasoning, as well as the ways that we act, and about the role that we ourselves can play in controlling pain. The therapy then goes on to teach a whole range of different coping strategies which can range from relaxation techniques which help to reduce muscle tension, alleviate emotional distress and distract patients from the sensations of pain, to how to pace activities and how to factor pleasant activities into their lives. In addition, it teaches them to challenge their own negative perceptions and thoughts about their pain and replace them with thoughts which better enable them to cope.

The final element of CBT is geared towards applying the coping skills and techniques that patients have learned to ever-wider ranges of daily situations. They learn how to develop problem-solving skills and plans to help them deal with flares-ups in their conditions, as well as other difficult situations that they might encounter, as well as how to monitor their own thoughts and behaviours to ensure continued benefit.

As you can see, CBT is very much a practically based therapy and one of the reasons that it works so well in the treatment of a range of different conditions is that it provides individuals with a set of tools that they can use for life. Once sufferers become aware of their own negative thinking and how this affects their behaviour, if they do find themselves starting off on a downward spiral they are able to recognise it straight away and, armed with the right techniques, they are able to correct their own course.

CBT can either be carried out on a one-on-one basis or in a group setting and your healthcare provider will be able to help you decide which is most appropriate for you.

21

Diet and Lifestyle

Even in an otherwise healthy person, a poor diet will eventually take its toll and cause a downturn in levels of general health. In someone who is suffering from any type of illness, a diet which is not balanced and which does not contain all of the nutrients that the body requires will again affect overall health and may aggravate the symptoms of the condition.

As I mentioned in Chapter 19, health food stores and internet sites advertise a whole range of dietary supplements which they claim can help with the symptoms of arthritis. In many cases there is no scientific evidence to support these claims and in some cases the supplements and diets which are recommended can even be harmful. In their attempts to find anything that might help with their conditions, however, a great many arthritis sufferers spend vast amounts of money on these products.

While there are people with arthritis who find that eliminating certain foodstuffs from their diets helps with their symptoms, as I said in Chapter 7, this may simply be because the individual has an intolerance or an allergy to particular foods anyway. Certainly there does not seem to be any scientific evidence to suggest that specific foods aggravate the symptoms of the condition and this is evidenced by the fact that no two arthritis patients seem to respond in the same way to the elimination of the same dietary elements.

Of course, for anyone with arthritis, arming the body with the right nutrients is vital to enable them to fight back against the disease and to stop them from succumbing to other additional illnesses. For sufferers who are overweight, however, diet takes on another level of importance, because of course obesity is one of the major risk factors for osteoarthritis of the knees and hips in particular, and in other forms of the disease excess weight also puts undue pressure on the joints as well as limiting mobility in itself. When you bear in mind that there is a four to five pound reduction in the stress placed on the knees for each pound of body weight lost, it is easy to see that even losing a few pounds can make a considerable difference to a sufferer's levels of pain and their overall quality of life.

Although the market is full of slimming products and so-called 'miracle diets', as many people who have tried these will know, what typically happens is that the weight just piles back on when they return to normal eating habits. In addition, these special treatments and diets are frequently unbalanced, leaving those who use them deficient in essential vitamins, minerals and other nutrients. The only real and healthy way to lose weight and keep it off, therefore, is simply by adjusting the amount and the type of food that you eat, as well as the amount of exercise that you do.

Eating a balanced diet which contains all of the essential nutrients is absolutely key to maintaining health and Arthritis Research UK recommends a diet which includes all of the following food groups in the following proportions:

- Fruits and vegetables (with the exception of potatoes) – one-third of diet by weight
- Starchy foods such as bread, potatoes, pasta and cereals – one-third of diet by weight
- Dairy products, including milk, cheese and yoghurt, but not cream or butter – one-sixth of diet by weight
- Foods containing protein such as fish, meat, eggs, pulses and soya products – one-eighth of diet by weight
- Occasional fatty or sugary foods such as cakes, butter, cream, ice-cream and sweets

The fats and oils which are contained in our food and which are used to cook it play an extremely important role in terms of overall health and weight loss or gain. The main types of fat are:

- Saturated fats, which come from meat and dairy products

- Polyunsaturated fats, which are contained in sunflower oil, corn oil and most nut oils, and
- Monounsaturated fats, which are found in olive and canola oils

Of these three types, monounsaturated fats are the ones which should make up the largest proportion of the fats that we eat, with polyunsaturated fats being used only in moderation and saturated fats being least used.

Although it is tempting to think of any kind of fat in our diets as bad, this is not in fact the case. We need the essential fatty acids omega-6 and omega-3 in order to remain healthy, but as our bodies cannot produce these, they have to be incorporated into our diet in the right proportions through certain types of foods. The ratio of omega-6 to omega-3 years ago was thought to be around 1:1 and this is still considered to be ideal, but nowadays the diets that many people eat tend to be weighted heavily towards sunflower, corn, soy and other types of oil which are rich in omega-6 but contain no omega-3. In fact, the amount of omega-6 that most people consume now is thought to be anywhere between 20 and 50 times the amount of omega-3 and, as the latter is what helps to protect our bodies from heart disease, depression, certain types of cancer, fibromyalgia and arthritis, it is small wonder that we are seeing so many more cases of these illnesses.

Unlike omega-6, which comes from a number of different sources, omega-3 is only found in fish oil and a handful of other foodstuffs, although of course omega-3 capsules are widely available and can be used as a supplement. As noted in Chapter 19, fish oil capsules are one of the very few dietary supplements which have been shown to be genuinely beneficial for rheumatoid arthritis, as well as for other inflammatory types of the disease, and in addition these help to protect against heart disease.

When buying or preparing foods, there are several things that you can do to cut down your intake of unhealthy fats, including by:

- Checking the labels of any prepared foodstuffs that you buy. Many of these, such as biscuits, cakes, chocolate and savoury snacks contain unexpectedly high levels of fat

- Choosing lean cuts of meat and trimming off any excess fat or, better still, opting for fish and poultry
- Choosing low-fat dairy products such as skimmed or semi-skimmed milk, low-fat cheese and yoghurt
- Using olive oil in preference to sunflower, corn or nut oils
- Using margarines containing olive oil or soya
- Grilling food in preference to frying. If you do enjoy the occasional fry-up, then use just a small amount of olive oil

Although, as I have said, ideally it is better to ensure a healthy, balanced diet which includes all of the food groups indicated earlier, some people who suffer from arthritis have found it to be beneficial to switch to a vegetarian or vegan diet. If this is something that you want to consider, then be sure to discuss it with your healthcare practitioner or the nutritionist who is part of your pain management team first, as these diets may not be suitable for everyone and do need to be used carefully to ensure that the body still receives the right quantities of all the essential nutrients.

While maintaining a proper balanced diet is essential for everyone, when it comes to body weight, it is of course important to know whether you sit within the normal range as opposed to being overweight or underweight. This can be determined quickly and easily by calculating your body mass index (BMI) using the following formula:

Weight in kilograms ÷ height in metres squared

Thus, if your height is 1.67m and your weight is 95kgs, the calculation would look like this:

$$1.67 \times 1.67 = 2.78$$
$$95 \div 2.78 = 34.17$$

As the ideal range for BMI for most people is between 18.5 and 25, a score of 34.17 would indicate being seriously overweight.

Alcohol

Studies in relation to alcohol consumption generally have shown conflicting results, although most tend to indicate that moderate amounts of beer, wine or spirits can help to reduce a person's risk of heart disease and stroke. What about the effects of alcohol on arthritis sufferers though? Does it help the condition or make it worse?

A study which was conducted by the University of Sheffield, the results of which were published in 2010, showed that those rheumatoid arthritis sufferers who had drunk alcohol most frequently throughout a one month period prior to the start of the study suffered less joint pain, swelling and disability than those who had drunk no alcohol at all or who had only drunk infrequently. In addition, X-rays showed less damage to the joints and blood tests indicated less inflammation. Although the reasons for this are by no means fully understood, the consultant rheumatologist who led the study was reported as saying that there is some evidence to suggest that alcohol suppresses the activity of the immune system and that the anti-inflammatory and analgesic effects of alcohol may reduce the severity of symptoms. What is important to note here, however, is that none of the patients who took part in this research consumed more than the recommended limit of 10 units per week.

This, of course, was just one study and should in no way be considered as a signal for arthritis sufferers to take up drinking. The issue of alcohol is a complex one and there are some very important issues which those with arthritis need to take into consideration.

- Although alcohol may help to dull pain, it can also affect our sense of judgement and lead us to take risks that we might not normally take or to extend our normal limits. A few drinks might, for example, make you feel able to dance the night away, but you could be left feeling the effects for days afterwards.

- Drinking alcohol affects the sense of co-ordination, making trips and falls more likely and possibly causing further damage to already painful joints.

- Mixing alcohol with medications is not only inadvisable, but in some cases it can be downright dangerous. Not only is there the chance that the effect of the alcohol could be doubled, but there is also a risk of increased side effects. In some cases, the combination of alcohol and medications such as methotrexate can cause liver damage.

■ Some reports suggest that alcohol can increase the risk of osteoporosis.

■ Alcohol is a known risk factor for gout.

■ Alcohol contains empty calories and can lead to weight gain.

■ Self-medicating with alcohol can lead to serious addiction problems.

Generally speaking, unless drinking alcohol is contraindicated because of the medications that you are taking or because of other health concerns, a glass or two of your favourite beverage on the odd occasion probably will not cause any harm. Moderation, however, is very much the watchword where alcohol is concerned and under no circumstances is it wise to exceed the recommended daily or weekly limits. In addition, it is worth remembering that other studies have shown that drinking more than two alcoholic drinks per day can increase the risk of certain types of cancer, including cancer of the colon, breast cancer and cancers of the mouth and throat.

Smoking

Talking about quitting smoking to someone who has been smoking for years can sometimes be like waving a red flag in front of a bull, and many regular smokers will try to justify their habit in any way possible rather than face the pain of stopping. Even suggesting that they are more likely to die a horrible death from lung cancer or heart disease does not discourage them, because unless and until such time as these diseases present themselves, they are just 'things that happen to other people'.

Smokers take a lot of flack about their addiction, but often all this does is to raise their stress levels so that all they want to do is reach for another cigarette. In addition, in many cases little or no attempt is made to explain precisely how smoking can have detrimental effects on their bodies. If you are a smoker who is reading this book, however, you probably already have arthritis and so the disease that we are talking about is not one which only happens to other people – it happened to you. In fact, if you are a smoker and a sufferer of rheumatoid arthritis, your chances of developing the condition were twice as high as those of a non-smoker. Whichever type of arthritis you have though, smoking will affect the severity of your symptoms, make it harder for your body to heal itself, may render certain medications ineffective so that you experience greater suffering and may preclude you from benefitting from certain types of surgery which could vastly improve your quality of life.

Without going into complex medical explanations, several of the key ways in which smoking affects the body are as follows:

- Smoking reduces the amount of oxygen in the body. Oxygen is needed by all of the body's cells to convert food into energy. If insufficient oxygen reaches the muscles of the heart, this can cause damage and deterioration, and if the muscles of the body do not receive enough oxygen this results in pain and muscle fatigue
- Smoking causes the blood vessels to constrict which means that decreased levels of nutrients and oxygen reach the body's organs and bones, which in turn means that bones take longer to heal
- The toxins in cigarettes also hinder the body's healing processes. In cases of injury or when a person undergoes surgery, the delay in healing can leave the patient more susceptible to infection

Until or unless smoking is banned altogether, anyone of legal age can of course make up their own mind as to whether the 'benefits' outweigh the risks and it is certainly not my place to dictate that any smoker must quit. As a doctor, however, it is my duty to point out that if you wish to minimise the pain of your condition and improve your overall health and quality of life, then stopping smoking is in your own best interests.

Caring for Your Joints

For most people, the way in which they use their joints probably is not something that they spend much time thinking about. For someone whose joints have already been compromised by arthritis, however, there can often be a great deal of fear in terms of causing further damage.

Taking care of your joints, even when carrying out everyday tasks, is of course important, and so in this chapter I offer some tips to help minimise the risk of joint strains, stresses and injuries.

- Try to get down to and maintain the ideal body weight for your height. Any additional weight will only put more stress on your joints, especially your knees, hips, ankles, feet and back.

- Be sure to keep up with the exercises recommended to you by your physiotherapist or pain management specialist. Joints affected by arthritis can become unstable, but exercise helps to strengthen the muscles around them, so providing greater stability.

- Try to avoid standing or sitting in one position for too long so that your joints do not become stiff. If you do have to stand for any length of time, place one foot on a low stool to help with your posture. Wherever possible, alternate standing and sitting.

- Pay attention to which positions and movements make you feel stiff and sore and then tell your physiotherapist or occupational therapist so that he or she can recommend better and more efficient ways of using your body.

- Try to avoid awkward positions or movements which might strain your joints. Stop and think about the safest way to do something.

- Stand up straight without locking your knees. The taller and straighter you stand, the less pressure you will put on the larger, weight-bearing joints of your body.

- Pace your activities throughout the day and alternate periods of heavy activity with periods of rest.

- Avoid carrying out repetitive activities for prolonged periods of time.

- If pain and stiffness feel worse in the mornings, then schedule your activities so that the hardest tasks are left until later in the day.

- Where possible, try to rely on the larger, stronger joints rather than the smaller, weaker ones. If your arthritis affects your hands, wrists or elbows, for example, then try using your shoulders to push open doors or use a shoulder bag to carry shopping rather than a hand-held one.

- Rather than putting all of the strain on a single joint, think about how you can spread the load such as by using both hands to lift or carry items instead of just one.

- The tighter you grip things, the more strain is placed on the joints of your fingers, so try to hold items as loosely as possible. Do make sure though, that your grip is secure enough to avoid dropping things accidentally.

- Always be sure to use any specialised equipment that you have been provided with or which has been recommended to you, whether it be a wrist rest for use with a computer or a lumbar support belt to avoid back injuries when lifting.

- Always take extreme care if you are taking part in any activity that you have never tried before. Sometimes it can be difficult to judge whether joints or muscles are likely to take a pounding and if so, which ones. Take it slowly so that you have a chance to assess how your body will respond.

- Never be afraid to ask for help. No matter how big or small a task, if you do not think you can handle it safely alone, then ask someone to help you out.

Remember, your physiotherapist and occupational therapist will be able to help you with posture and movement, as well as with suggestions for simple adaptations to make your life easier and more comfortable.

23

How to Control Stress

Stress is the physical and emotional response to tensions and pressures and of course it is something that we all experience at various times in our lives to varying degrees. As with the pain of arthritis, just how each individual experiences stress and what they perceive to be a stressful situation varies from person to person, but certainly it is not only major life events which can cause a reaction. For some, the minor niggles that we all experience on a day-to-day basis, such as getting stuck in traffic jams, dealing with poor customer service or facing a deadline at work, can raise stress levels sky high, whereas for others such a response only comes with major events such as bereavement or job loss. There is no 'norm' as far as stress is concerned and everyone reacts differently to potentially stressful situations.

Of course, alongside the everyday stresses that we all have to deal with, people with arthritis and other chronic pain conditions have a whole host of other challenges and frustrations to face. Constant levels of pain, lack of mobility, fatigue and depression, not to mention lowered self-esteem, lack of self-confidence, poor self-image, issues of dependence, relationship problems, work issues and practical concerns around finances can all add enormously to the stress that they experience. When stress becomes an added burden though, and especially when it is unrelenting, it can have a negative impact on physical well-being, causing symptoms to become more severe and making it harder for the body to heal itself. In this way, a vicious cycle is set up in which the difficulties of living with the disease cause stress, which in turn causes muscle tension and flare-ups in pain and other symptoms, which in turn causes more stress. Breaking free of this cycle is therefore vital if the condition is to be managed effectively, which is one of the reasons why stress-handling and relaxation techniques form important parts of cognitive behavioural therapy.

Because stress can very easily lead to anxiety and depression, taking early action to deal with it is important and there is much that sufferers can do to help themselves in this regard. In the remainder of this chapter, therefore, I offer a number of useful tips for getting stress under control and making life feel more manageable.

1. Much of the stress which is directly caused by arthritis comes from fear of the disease itself, such as the fears surrounding long-term prognosis or how the condition will affect the sufferer's daily life. As you have begun to do by reading this book, educate yourself about the particular type of arthritis that you have been diagnosed with. Ask your pain management specialist about anything that you do not understand, communicate with other sufferers and read anything that you can lay your hands on. Do be careful to choose only reliable sources of information, however. In an unregulated environment such as the internet, there is much information which is written by laymen and those who are only interested in selling their own 'miracle cures' for the disease, and some of it is not only misleading but could be potentially dangerous.

2. Accepting a chronic pain condition is crucial in being able to deal with it effectively and in keeping stress at bay. The Serenity Prayer, which has been adopted by a number of 12-step programmes, but which is in fact useful for anyone, irrespective of their circumstances, can act as a huge reminder of what we can and cannot control in our lives. The prayer goes like this:

> God grant me the serenity
> to accept the things I cannot change,
> courage to change the things I can
> and wisdom to know the difference

Understand that although there is currently no cure for arthritis, there is a great deal that you can do to take your own situation in hand and to improve your own quality of life. Know which things you do have control over, concentrate on these and your levels of stress will recede.

3. Stress can begin to feel overwhelming, to the extent that it becomes impossible to know for sure precisely what is causing it. Sit down and really identify the sources of your stress so that you can be proactive in dealing with them.

4. Some of the things which cause stress are things that we can avoid. If there are certain people or situations which are adding to your stressful feelings, then think about whether you can steer clear of them. Remember too that what you take into your body can make a huge difference in terms of the severity of your symptoms, so aim to avoid foods which are unhealthy or which add to weight problems, as well as excess alcohol and smoking. Most of us are perfectly aware of when we are not treating our bodies kindly and this can lead to guilt and then to stress.

5. Make sure that your expectations of yourself and others are realistic. The fact is that you may not be able to accomplish things in the same way that you did previously, but that is okay. Even under normal circumstances we are none of us perfect, so be kind to yourself. Also, try to be understanding of the people around you, as they may also be having a difficult time dealing with your illness and suffering their own stresses. Trust that they are doing their best to help and support you in the ways that they can and be grateful for their efforts, otherwise frustration, resentment and stress are likely to build.

6. Life is complicated and filled with activity, all of which can add to feelings of stress. Do whatever you can to simplify your life, whether that means rearranging your home to make things easier or more accessible or getting into a routine so that life's ups and downs are evened out.

7. Think about how you manage your time. Rushing around to try and fit everything in is guaranteed to raise stress levels, so try and plan your activities in advance, remembering to allow yourself more time than you might have needed in the past to take

account of any mobility problems. Also, bear in mind that the aim should be to do things as efficiently as possible in order to conserve energy, so think about how you do things, as well as about the times of day when you feel most able to carry out your tasks.

8. As I mentioned previously, stress can quickly become an issue when our lives feel out of control, and a feeling of drifting or of getting nowhere can quickly raise anxiety levels. Counteract these feelings by setting short- and longer-term goals for yourself. Your arthritis might be life-altering, but it is not life-ending, so give yourself objectives to aim for and you will have the satisfaction of feeling that you are moving inexorably forwards.

9. Face up to practical issues such as financial problems, because otherwise these will simply eat away at you and rob you of your peace of mind. Although it might feel difficult to pick up the telephone and speak to the bank manager or credit card company, once you have discussed your circumstances and come to a manageable arrangement you will feel more in control and stress levels will drop.

10. When we feel stressed, we tend to fixate on problems so that they go round and round in our minds and we start to imagine the worst possible scenarios. Try learning the art of meditation to help relax body and mind, or lose yourself in a relaxation tape or some gentle, soothing music.

11. Another great way to escape from stressful feelings is to let yourself become totally absorbed in a favourite hobby or pastime. Activities which are peaceful but require concentration, such as drawing, painting or needlework can be excellent ways to forget your troubles for a while and unwind.

12. Take a relaxing bath when you feel stressed. Not only will the warm water help you to relax, but it will also help to relieve pain.

13. Sometimes the best way to deal with stress is simply to take some time out, away from the hustle and bustle. Either find a room in the house where you can just sit quietly and relax, or take yourself off on a solitary walk to clear your head.

14. Take time out to have fun with friends and family, and especially to indulge your sense of humour. Even simple things like playing

board games or watching your favourite comedy film or series on TV can really help to lift your spirits and push stress aside.

15. Learn when to say 'no'. Putting yourself under pressure by agreeing to do things that you do not feel up to will only lead to increased stress.

16. Share what you are thinking and feeling with others. Try not to nag and complain about symptoms, as this is only likely to raise your stress levels rather than reduce them. Instead, talk about your underlying fears and worries and they will instantly become less frightening. Reach out to friends or family members, or communicate with other sufferers through one of the excellent online or offline arthritis support services.

17. No-one likes to feel dependent on others, but if there are genuinely times when you need help, then ask for it. People are not mind readers and they do not always spot when we are feeling overwhelmed by stress and nor do they necessarily know what they can do to help. Helping others makes us feel good and the chances are that your loved ones will welcome the opportunity to lend a hand, rather than feeling helpless.

18. Exercise is not only an excellent way to manage stress, because it promotes the release of the body's feel-good hormones, but of course it also increases your overall physical fitness and makes you more mentally alert.

19. Try writing about the things which make you feel stressed. Writing can be a great way to get feelings out into the open instead of letting them go round and round inside you, and often it can help solutions to appear quite unexpectedly before you. Remember that you do not have to show your writing to another soul, so go ahead and let it all out.

20. If stress starts to get the better of you and you feel that you are being overtaken by anxiety or depression, never turn to alcohol or illicit drugs for comfort as these will only create more problems and could ultimately cause you additional lifelong suffering. Instead, talk to your healthcare practitioner who may be able to prescribe appropriate antidepressant medication or recommend therapy to help you deal with it.

Part IV

Understanding Medico-Legal Implications

24

Personal Injury Claims and Arthritis

As you will have seen from Chapter 3 of this book, the causes and triggers of arthritis are many and in some cases they are not particularly well understood. In some cases, autoimmune disorders are almost certainly at the root of the disease, whereas in others genetic and other factors coupled with the general wear and tear on the body may play a part in its development.

In many cases of arthritis, patients are able to trace the onset of their condition back to an earlier accident or injury, and sometimes this is even true of the autoimmune forms of the disease such as rheumatoid arthritis. In Chapter 3, I mentioned the famous example of former Arsenal goalkeeper Bob Wilson and his struggle with osteoarthritis after years of punishing injuries during his time as a footballer, and indeed sporting injuries do account for a good number of cases of arthritis. Sometimes, however, the types of accidents and injuries which lead to the development of the disease are not ones which come about through deliberate lifestyle choices such as the hobbies and pastimes that we choose to take part in, but rather through the negligence of others. Of course, in the case of Bob Wilson and other professional sportspeople and athletes, their sport is more than just a hobby, but the injuries which they sustain as a result could hardly be considered to be the result of any negligence on the part of their employers, but are simply occupational hazards.

Some put the figure for post-traumatic arthritis (arthritis caused by accident or injury) at as high as 10% of all cases. While many of these, of course, are simply the result of trips or falls in which there is no negligence on the part of another, in other cases this is not so. Employers who fail to provide appropriate training or equipment for their workers, for example, or drivers who cause motoring accidents might be considered to be negligent, and where this is the case, the victim of the accident may be able to make a rightful claim against them and be entitled to an appropriate amount of compensation. Even slips or falls which are caused by a company's or local authority's failure to mop up spills on the floor of a shop or to fix broken paving slabs can form the basis of a personal injury claim.

Of course, the trouble with arthritis in relation to earlier accidents and injuries is that often the disease does not show itself until a long while afterwards, in some cases years later. By the time it does develop, the victim either does not make any connection between the two events or considers it too late to make any kind of claim against the negligent party. Although, generally speaking, it is quite true that personal injury claims must be made within three years of the accident, in cases where the true nature of the injury did not become apparent until much later, this deadline can, however, sometimes be extended.

The law in relation to personal injury claims permits someone who has suffered an accident or injury through the fault of another person or organisation to seek damages for pain and suffering, as well as to reimburse them for any expenses, such as medical fees, and losses, including any loss of earnings that the individual may have had to suffer. If such a claim is made, then the claimant (or the plaintiff as he or she is known) is represented by a solicitor whose job it is to prove the liability of the other party (the defendant) and to persuade the compensator, which is usually an insurance company, to make an appropriate award for damages. The compensator, of course, also has a legal representative, and his or her aim is to prove that the client was not guilty of negligence, or at the very least to minimise the amount of compensation which is paid out.

In order for the claimant's lawyer to be able to prove that arthritis developed as a direct result of the other party's negligence, the claimant needs to be assessed by a medical expert who specialises in the condition. Once this expert has prepared his or her report and provided it to the solicitor, the insurer then has a specified amount of time in which to accept or deny liability and, if liability is accepted, the two sides would then negotiate a mutually acceptable settlement. In most cases where liability is accepted, any costs associated with the claim are paid by the defendant's insurer and not by the claimant him or herself.

As you might imagine, personal injury claims are adversarial in nature. Clearly, the defendant's insurer wants to avoid having to pay out compensation, but at the same time the plaintiff's solicitor is fighting to achieve an appropriate amount of compensation on behalf of the claimant, whose quality of life may have been severely affected as the result of the other party's negligence. It is often because of the adversarial nature of these cases that many people are discouraged from pursuing a claim, when in fact they might have a very good case.

One of the important things to know about personal injury claims is that they work quite differently from the criminal cases that most of us are more familiar with. In the latter, of course, the lawyer for the prosecution has to prove 'beyond reasonable doubt' that the defendant is guilty if he or she is to win the case. Where personal injury claims are concerned, however, the burden of proof is quite different. In these cases, which come under the area of civil rather than criminal law, the burden of proof is on the balance of probabilities, so that all the claimant's solicitor has to demonstrate is that, on balance, the plaintiff's injuries were more likely to have been caused by the other party's negligence than not.

Of course, even though cases involving personal injury claims do not have to be absolutely watertight in the same way as criminal cases, they can still be difficult, although by no means impossible to win. Much depends on the experience of the plaintiff's solicitor in dealing with such cases, and also the evidence of the medical expert is absolutely crucial in determining the outcome of the case. Although arthritis is a very common disease, because there is much about it which is not understood by many in the medical profession, solicitors who act on the behalf of plaintiff's often recommend that he or she secures the services of a medico-legal expert who is highly experienced in the disease itself, as well as in its relationship with traumatic injuries. Such experts are typically much more successful, not only in terms of showing that the balance of probability falls in favour of the plaintiff, but also in securing higher levels of compensation.

25

Medico-Legal Experts and Personal Injury Solicitors

When it comes to choosing a medical expert to represent you in a personal injury claim, there are of course a great many practitioners who are very knowledgeable in the field of arthritis. Not all, however, are best equipped or experienced to be able to present their evidence in a sufficiently convincing way to secure a claim. A medico-legal expert, on the other hand, possesses both the medical skills and knowledge to make an expert clinical assessment of the patient and the requisite legal knowledge to be able to present his or her findings in a way which is acceptable in a legal sense and convincing enough to make winning the case more likely.

As I explained in the previous chapter, once a medical expert has assessed your case, he or she will then compile a full report of your medical status which is provided to your solicitor. These reports do, of course, vary in terms of their contents and how thorough they are depending upon the medical expert that you choose. A good medico-legal expert who works in a multidisciplinary environment and has direct access to the expert opinions of a range of specialists from different backgrounds, however, will be able to provide you with a fully comprehensive report which builds a strong case for your claim. At the London Pain Clinic, for example, we provide a full medico-legal report which contains the following:

1. Details
2. Content
3. Introduction

4. Methodology
5. History
6. Examination
7. Opinion
8. Prognosis
9. Medico-legal declaration
10. Curriculum Vitae

In addition, wherever possible, the report will conclude with our recommendations for treatment.

Actually, this final point raises another extremely important role of a medico-legal expert, because of course securing compensation for a personal injury is not the only concern if you now find yourself faced with living with chronic arthritis. As we have seen throughout the course of this book, chronic arthritis has the potential to have devastating impacts on the sufferer's quality of life and so diagnosing the condition quickly, treating it appropriately using a range of different techniques and teaching the individual how to manage the condition successfully are all vital if any sense of normality and a good quality of life are to be restored and maintained. In the hands of a good medico-legal expert, not only are the chances of a successful personal injury claim greatly enhanced, but the claimant also benefits from the very best ongoing medical care.

As I mentioned earlier, one of the things which discourages many people from pursuing a personal injury claim is that they fear that their chances of winning are likely to be slim. Another reason though, is because they fear that the whole process is likely to be extremely costly, and after having perhaps had to pay out for expensive medical costs already, the prospect of then having to stump up for legal fees is not something that most could consider, especially as legal aid is not available in most cases involving personal injury. Many personal injury solicitors nowadays, however, work on a 'no win no fee' basis, which means that the claimant does not have to pay for the legal costs associated with the case unless the case is won. Even if the case is won, however, it is the defendant's side which pays the solicitor's fees, and normally any court fees and medical report costs too. Obviously, if a solicitor is going to take on a case on such a basis, he or she will need to feel reasonably assured of winning, which is another reason why it is advisable to choose a good medico-legal representative who is able to provide the strongest medical evidence to support the claim.

As well as fighting the claim on your behalf and achieving the highest possible level of compensation, another important role which is played by your legal representative is in securing interim payments. You may, for example, already have had to pay for medical expenses or your earning capability may have been affected by your condition, leaving you out of pocket. Because the negotiations in relation to personal injury claims can sometimes drag on, in cases where the defendant admits liability but a settlement figure is yet to be determined, your solicitor may be able to secure part of your compensation in the form of one or more interim payments to help to alleviate any financial burden or suffering that you might be experiencing in the meantime. You could, for example, use an interim payment to pay medical costs or to have any necessary adaptations made to your home to make your life easier.

The amount of the interim payment will, of course, depend on your circumstances and it cannot exceed what would be considered a 'reasonable proportion' of the final expected payout. When the case is concluded, the total amount of any interim payments is deducted from the overall agreed amount of compensation.

Conclusion

Arthritis affects hundreds of millions of people around the world and, as life expectancies rise, so the number of people who are diagnosed with the condition is likely to keep on growing. As we have seen though, far from being the 'old people's disease' that many consider it to be, arthritis in its many forms is a disease which can strike at any time. Not only the elderly, but also children, adolescents and those in the prime of their lives can suddenly find themselves faced with the prospect of a lifetime of pain and restricted mobility when the condition is diagnosed.

Although it is easy to think of arthritis as being a strictly physiological illness, like so many other chronic pain conditions it is one whose effects extend far beyond its physical symptoms. Even once the initial shock of being diagnosed with the disease has worn off, each new day brings with it more and more examples of the limitations which are suddenly placed on sufferers' lives and, as their worlds begin to feel as if they are closing in, so they sink further and further into emotional and psychological despair.

For those on the outside, it can be hard to imagine the utter devastation that a chronic pain condition can cause. Diseases such as arthritis have the potential to test relationships to the limits, to impact enormously on home, family, work and social lives and ultimately to make sufferers feel robbed of their choices and of any semblance of a normal life. Even many doctors though, continue to treat arthritis as a simple physical disease without taking into account the much more widespread impacts that it typically has on patients' lives.

Arthritis is a complex disease, but what I hope you will have understood from this book is that it does not have to be one which destroys your quality of life. By approaching your situation with a positive frame of mind and with determination and commitment, you can take control of the disease, instead of letting the disease control you. With an open mind, greater awareness and the willingness to explore new avenues, anyone of any age can minimise the effects of this potentially debilitating condition and live a happy and successful life which is relatively free of pain or even completely pain free.

Simplistic approaches to arthritis which only deal with physical symptoms or which only treat those symptoms with traditional pharmaceutical medications cause unnecessary suffering to millions of people who have been diagnosed with the disease. Research has shown conclusively time and time again that the key to tackling chronic pain conditions effectively is by treating the person, not just the disease in isolation. After all, you are not your disease. You are a unique individual with your own unique set of thoughts, feelings, perceptions, experiences and needs, and so it is not hard to see how a multidisciplinary treatment programme which is tailor-made to suit your particular circumstances and which takes all of these things into account can only be more effective than a standard approach which merely sees you labelled as another arthritis patient.

Being diagnosed with arthritis does not have to mean the beginning of the end. You can take back the control of your own life and whether you have only recently been diagnosed with the disease or have been living with it for many years, I sincerely hope that this book has helped to demonstrate how that is possible and the options which are available to you.

If there is any other information, advice or support that I can offer, then please do not hesitate to contact me. In the meantime, all that remains is to wish you everything good in life and my very best wishes!

Dr Christopher Jenner MB BS, FCRA
London Pain Clinic
www.londonpainclinic.com

Index

Fibromyalgia and Myofascial Pain Syndrome
A practical guide to getting on with your life

Dr Chris Jenner

There really is life after being diagnosed with fibromyalgia or myofascial pain syndrome . . . and yours starts here.

The lack of knowledge which surrounds two of the most prevalent illnesses in the world today means that they can often go undiagnosed and untreated for years, during which time both the mental and physical condition of sufferers can deteriorate considerably.

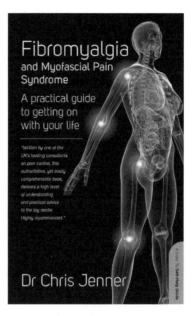

With the right care, there is much that can be done to help anyone with these conditions to improve their quality of life dramatically. The first step towards that is by doing precisely what you are doing now, educating yourself.

Within the covers of this book, you will find an easy-to-read and practical guide to dealing with fibromyalgia and myofascial pain. Dr Chris Jenner takes a straightforward and down-to-earth look at what these two conditions are about; how they might affect different aspects of your life; what your options are; and how you can get on with your life.

ISBN 978-1-84528-467-1

Neck and Back Pain
A practical guide to getting on with your life

Dr Chris Jenner

Far from just being the curse of the elderly, neck and back pain affects the majority of the adult population at some point in their lives, as well as huge numbers of children and adolescents. Even in chronic cases, however, it does not have to mean the end of life as you once knew it. With the knowledge contained in this book and the right care, you *can* regain control and live a happy and productive life.

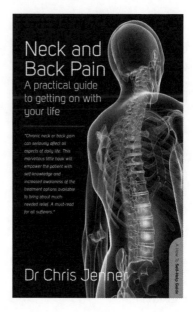

In his reassuringly down-to-earth guide, Dr Chris Jenner describes the many causes of neck and back pain in easily understood laymen's terms. He then explores what it means to live with neck and back conditions in a practical sense, sets out your treatment options, and advises on how you can very greatly reduce your levels of pain and increase your quality of life.

ISBN 978-1-84528-468-8